MEDICAL DEVICES FOR RESPIRATORY DYSFUNCTION:

PRINCIPLES AND MODELING OF CONTINUOUS POSITIVE AIRWAY PRESSURE (CPAP)

Author

Ahmed M. Al-Jumaily
Institute of Biomedical Technologies
Auckland University of Technology

Contributing Author

Prasika I. Reddy
Institute of Biomedical Technologies
Auckland University of Technology

ASME PRESS

ASME Press books are available at special quantity discounts to use as premiums or for use in corporate training programs. For more information, contact Special Sales at infocentral@asme.org

Library of Congress Cataloging-in-Publication Data

Al-Jumaily, Ahmed.
Medical devices for respiratory dysfunction : principles and modeling of continuous positive airway pressure (CPAP) devices / Ahmed M. Al-Jumaily ; contributing author, Prasika I. Reddy.
p. ; cm.
Includes bibliographical references.
ISBN 978-0-7918-5977-3
I. Reddy, Prasika I. II. Title.
[DNLM: 1. Continuous Positive Airway Pressure--instrumentation. 2. Biomedical Engineering--methods. 3. Respiration Disorders--therapy. 4. Sleep Apnea, Obstructive--therapy. WF 145]

616.20028'4--dc23

2011035639

TABLE OF CONTENTS

ABOUT THE AUTHOR

Professor Ahmed Al-Jumaily holds a Ph.D. and M.Sc. from Ohio State University, Columbus, OH, and a B.Sc. from the University of Baghdad, Iraq (all in Mechanical Engineering). He has 33 years of teaching and research experience at two American universities, four Middle Eastern universities, and the Auckland University of Technology (AUT). He is a Fellow member of the American Society of Mechanical Engineers, as well as a member of the Acoustical Society of America, American Engineering Education, International Society of Optical Engineering, International Institute of Acoustics and Vibration, and Institute of Professional Engineers New Zealand. He is also a registered professional engineer. He has supervised more than 90 postgraduate students in biomechanics, mechanical vibrations, acoustics, smart polymers, medical devices, and system dynamics and control. He has published more than 250 papers in international journals and conference proceedings, and has acted as a reviewer for several international journals. Also, he has edited two ASME books on vibration and acoustics in biomedical applications. As the director of the Engineering Research Institute and then the Institute of Biomedical Technologies of AUT for the last 12 years, he has established very strong industrial research links with many major medical device companies in New Zealand and the United States. Al-Jumaily's perspective of academic engineering research is that industrial research is a "must" to minimize the gap between academia and the industry.

PREFACE

This book introduces the reader to the basic principles of operation, development, and modeling of positive airway pressure therapy devices with an emphasis on Continuous Positive Airway Pressure (CPAP) devices. It includes updated literature reviews on the state of the art of these devices, including functionality and modeling. The book elaborates on two of the most prevalent respiratory dysfunctions, Obstructive Sleep Apnea (OSA) and Respiratory Distress Syndrome (RDS), with an emphasis on the use of CPAP systems to manage these respiratory disorders. It reflects more than 10 years of development, design, modeling, and improvement using electromechanical engineering principles to serve the medical community.

The book consists of an introductory chapter and two sections. Each one of the chapters in these sections is designed to be a stand-alone chapter that can potentially be used in an engineering modeling course. The introductory chapter presents some modeling concepts and their pros and cons, with emphasis on medical therapy device applications. The chapter also introduces a new concept of "Talkative Models," which can be used to assess medical device performance as these devices are applied during a therapy process.

Section One consists of six chapters, which focus on CPAP devices for OSA treatment. The first chapter in this section, i.e., Chapter 2 in the book, covers basic principles and current treatments of OSA. It presents definitions and an overview of OSA and the related literature, as well as elaborates on various methods of treatment. Chapter 3 demonstrates how modeling techniques can be applied to predict the performance of a prototype CPAP system. The system is described in terms of governing equations of the individual components using a lumped parameter approach, and then modeled in Simulink™ within the Matlab™ environment. The manner in which the governing equations can be detailed through the use of block diagrams within Simulink™ is demonstrated. Dynamic testing for the purpose of model verification is then illustrated to the reader. An example of how such a model can then be used for further product development is given by using it to evaluate the specifications of an improved air delivery unit. The need for modeling humidification and the types of humidifiers using a lumped parameter approach with model validation is presented in Chapter 4. While Chapter 5 covers the development of a control scheme to enable the regulation of a constant nasal mask pressure during CPAP therapy throughout a patient's breathing cycle, Chapter 6 presents a brief overview of the different types of masks used in CPAP delivery and an introduction to the importance of controlling carbon dioxide and condensation levels in the mask. This chapter also shows how fluid mechanics and thermodynamics can be used to model flow and condensation in a typical nasal mask. A computation fluid dynamics (CFD) approach to modeling condensation in the mask is also described when there is a need to take into account geometric complexity, flow direction, and temperature distribution.

Section Two consists of three chapters on RDS. The first chapter is Chapter 7 in the book. It provides an introduction and overview of RDS, and describes traditional surfactant and ventilation therapies, along with more current techniques that use pressure oscillations. In particular, the Bubble CPAP system is elaborated on, along with clinical studies from the literature that outline the benefits of its use to treat RDS. Chapter 8 provides a description of the various components of a Bubble CPAP system, before embarking on a lumped parameter modeling approach, where basic laws of physics and empirical relationships are applied to generate mathematical models of individual components. It also presents a description of how to create an overall computational model of the system in Simulink™ within the Matlab™ environment. The process of validating the model with experimental data is elaborated on with the aim of producing a model that can be used for clinical and engineering trials. The last chapter, Chapter 9, provides an introduction to the structure, function, and mechanics of the respiratory system before proceeding to discuss existing models in the literature that have been developed to answer a variety of questions on respiratory performance. The procedure of developing a validated lumped parameter mathematical model of a non-linear biological system such as the lung is described, and its implementation in the Simulink™ environment is also elaborated on. Using the "Talkative Models" concept introduced in Chapter 1, the manner in which such a model can be integrated with a model of a respiratory device to determine the effect of device operation on respiratory performance is illustrated.

The content and format of this book have been designed to benefit a variety of audiences, including:

1. Academic educators teaching upper-level graduate courses in Biomedical Engineering.
2. Graduate and undergraduate students in biomedical, electrical, and mechanical engineering wanting to learn about modeling therapeutic devices and techniques and how those models can be used to assess the performance of these devices.

3. Researchers interested in learning relevant significant principles, theory, modeling, experimental, and clinical applications of biomedical systems.
4. Medical practitioners who are involved in using therapeutic techniques.
5. Industrial professionals wishing to understand the fundamentals and applications of lung therapy devices with a focus on CPAP devices.
6. Medical device manufacturing companies interested in expedient procedures for device analyses and development.

This book presents well-established modeling methods as applied to medical devices. The author's main contributions have been to the ways in which these methods are fine-tuned for uses related to medical therapy devices. I am thus indebted to the authors and postgraduate students whose works were gleaned (with appropriate references to the original publications) for this book to be developed.

AUTHOR'S INTRODUCTION

Applications of engineering principles for therapy devices are not available under one umbrella; they are scattered in various research articles and limited book chapters. This makes it difficult for the reader to access lung therapy devices in one ready-made volume. To achieve this goal, this book provides updated material on the subject: It gives the basic principles of these devices and explains how engineering modeling is used to improve, develop, and optimize these devices.

This book bridges the gap between academia and the industry in the area of biomedical devices and methodologies. It compiles experimental, theoretical, and computational methods applied to the medical devices under one roof. This is the first book that brings together engineering principles as applied to Lung Therapy Devices. Information from the classroom and the industry are brought together to the expanding field of biomedical devices.

This book summarizes more than 10 years of research and development that I have conducted with my postgraduate students. Each chapter stands alone and summarizes a complete project, which is further detailed in the thesis cited as the main reference for that chapter. In this way, I would like to acknowledge the contributions of all students whose theses are used as the main reference materials for this book. I would also like to acknowledge the effort of my student and colleague, co-author Dr. Prasika I. Reddy, who has helped in putting together parts of the book. Further, I would like to extend my thanks to my student and assistant Meha Mathur for helping to revise parts of the book, as well as an ex-colleague and friend David Dodd for the final proof-reading of the book.

The author hopes that the readers will find this book a valuable asset in keeping themselves abreast of the latest techniques in the beneficial system modeling approach applications for lung supportive devices. This book will appeal not only to fellow researchers, but also to practitioners, lecturers, and students of engineering and medicine as well as to medical device industry personnel.

The author's wish is that this book will interest and intrigue its readers to promote further useful modeling applications for medical devices, and render those modeling techniques as tools for computer simulations, which can be the base for a "Virtual Lab" to test the performance of those devices. This is a very powerful and economic approach to improving and developing those devices. It will minimize the trial-and-error processes that are currently used by many industries and reduce the risk of costly design changes.

Ahmed Al-Jumaily
Institute of Biomedical Technologies
Auckland University of Technology
Auckland, New Zealand

INTRODUCTION

Chapter 1

MODELING CONCEPTS

This chapter discusses the mathematical modeling process and how it can be an effective tool in developing a virtual lab of simulation for medical devices, with lung therapy devices in particular. The chapter introduces the concept of "Talkative Models" in biomedical applications. The discussion includes some criteria for selecting "Talkative Models": conditions imposed on the interfaces between the models; requirements of biological and medical device models; performance criterion; and a typical case study that applies the model of a Bubble continuous positive airway pressure (CPAP) device to lung models that represent lungs with respiratory distress syndrome (RDS) to assess device performance.

1.1 MATHEMATICAL MODELING

Engineers and scientists have been inspired by mathematics as a tool to analyze, explain, and validate their hypotheses and theories. Unfortunately, a common perception among people, including some educators, is that mathematics is a "bunch" of equations which are used to explore mathematical applications and train students. Traditional engineering on the other hand is defined as the application of science and mathematics by which the properties of matter and the sources of energy in nature are made useful to people. However, with the expansion of the engineering discipline and the evolution of new types of engineering such as biomedical engineering, this definition may be reformulated to state that "inspired by the laws of physics, mathematics is used as a translator to convert nature's resources to a product or to study a phenomenon (phenomena) or a criterion (criteria)."

In fact, engineers use mathematics as a tool to convert science and related theories to numbers, design charts, and figures where the design and manufacturing of various systems and components are developed.

These laws of physics include but are not limited to those governing mechanics, electricity, magnetism, thermodynamics, acoustics, etc. With these basic thoughts, the question of why engineers and scientists put so much emphasis on mathematics may be decided. This may be answered by the fact that:

- Mathematics is a tool that translates theories to the industrial world.
- It converts real systems of interest into models that can be analyzed and tested on a piece of paper.
- With the current advancement in computational methods, computers make mathematics a valuable tool to convert real systems into virtual systems on the computer.

In brief, mathematics in terms of what is called "engineering modeling" converts physical laws into a research methodology. The next question to ask is "Why model?" This is because modeling can:

- Simulate a system and a process for assessment or understanding.
- Change a realistic system to a system that can be dealt with by the touch of a button.
- Reduce the process of experimental trial and error to a minimum.
- Investigate system performance at varied system parameters before it is built.
- Obtain specifications and dimensions for the system to help the design process.

Although the process of accurate modeling requires experience in addition to knowledge in the area of modeling, it does save time, effort, and cost in achieving the final design goals. In a broad sense, the accuracy of modeling depends on the nature of the application. However, the modeling process leads to several beneficial outcomes which mean that:

- A real system can be studied for improvement, modifications, and/or optimization without subjecting it to change or damage.
- Through mathematical modeling a virtual laboratory can be developed on the computer for optimization, design, analysis, etc.
- System parameters can easily be varied to investigate the system behavior under these changes.
- From the developed model, various specifications can be obtained for the system to be used in design, development, and manufacturing.

With all the experience to date in modeling, its reliability is still questioned by many. However, the pace of technological change drives industries to implement modeling (otherwise they may fall behind competitors). Advanced and complex industries such as the aircraft, submarine, and space industries have produced good and reliable models for their current technologies. Further, even if modeling is not a perfect process, it definitely helps in assessing trends, behaviors, and performance.

With all these facts about modeling, many difficulties are faced within industry in terms of understanding the advantages of modeling. This may be attributed to the fact that many of the companies believe in hands-on improvements only, since they lack experience in modeling and its "know-how." Some consider it an academic or "theoretical" approach and of no interest to them, and some companies have no interest in spending money on such a "luxury."

However, a careful yet confident approach may convince those industries to implement modeling. This may be achieved by:

- Introducing the idea to them.
- Convincing them that it is workable.
- Giving them some incentives as to what they can gain from it.
- Helping them find financial resources.
- Bringing the classroom to a practical environment.
- Keeping academic staff updated on what local industries require.
- Serving the industries with top-level qualified people in the country.

1.2 TALKATIVE MODELS

The devices and components of a dynamic system communicate with each other by some sort of energy type signals. Those signals have to be of the same type before they can be clearly understood and an action taken by the next component or element. For example, if the transmitted signal is of an electrical nature, both of the connected elements must understand the electrical signal or a converter must be used to change the signal to the same form of the receiving signal. If the type of signal is considered a language of communication between these elements/devices, it can be assumed that those devices "talk" to each other. The word "talk" is used to imply communication. Thus, the term "Talkative Devices" implies devices or elements that can communicate with each other to achieve certain goals or objectives.

Talkative Models can talk or communicate with each other to assess the performance of a system or a device (see Figure 1-1). This kind of model is very useful in many applications, especially biomedical ones. The context of their application is wide; however, at this instance the focus is on therapeutic devices such as those used to overcome breathing difficulties.

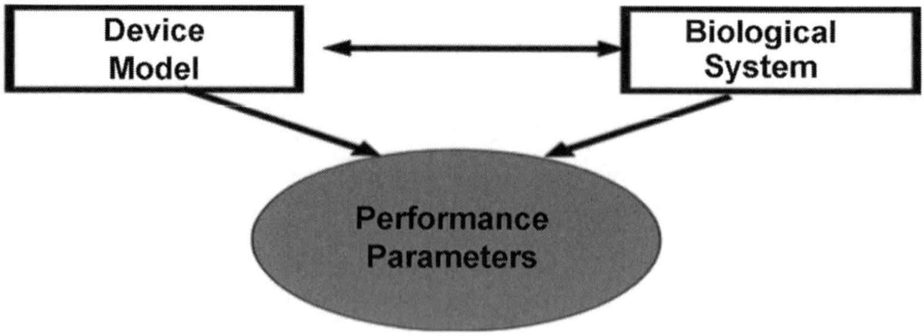

Figure 1-1. Device and biological system with common assessment parameters

It is possible to build a wide range of models for any particular system; however, specific limitations have to be set to develop functional models, namely models that have to achieve specific functions. For example, there are a variety of models for the lung. Some of them are too hypothetical while others are built to investigate a specific phenomenon or a process. Each of these models is built with certain objectives in mind. If, for example, the interest is in studying lung performance under obstructive sleep apnea (OSA), the objective of developing a model would be to assess the lung performance under various pressure and air supply conditions. The use of this model would be to specify functions that can show how effective a particular therapy is in overcoming the ailment. On the other hand, a model needs to be developed for the device that helps the lung to overcome the apnea. For example, in this case, a model of the CPAP device is developed with the objective of connecting this model to the lung model to determine performance criteria for the lung and/or the device. What would happen to the lung performance if one dimension or feature of the device is changed? If the device is misused, how would the lung respond?

Based on the common understanding of modeling, if the two models are developed for assessing the performance of a device under particular OSA conditions, those two models must be able to communicate with each other. The language of communication depends on the kind of energy exchange between the two systems; mathematics is still the core of most of the communication process. However, some conditions have to be imposed on the two models, such as:

- The models must be functional models that can be used as tools for any type of engineering evaluation or for the device.
- The models can be used as a tool in the everyday, real engineering environment.
- The models can be linked to bench and physiological testing to develop a virtual lab environment.

1.3 PARAMETER/MODEL REQUIREMENTS

The parameter of assessment represents variables that can be used to quantify measurements that can be made to assess the performance of the respiratory system and/or the biological system for which the device is used. These parameters should be:

- Capable of describing the mechanical response of the device and the biological system.
- Easily conceptualized and appreciated by clinicians.
- Non-invasively measured in experiments and practice.

In order to best explain this process, consider the following example:

Example: A model is to be built to assess the performance of a Bubble CPAP device as it is applied to RDS (see chapter 9 for details).

Purpose: The purpose of the mathematical model is to support clinical studies and identify mechanisms of improvement due to the device.

Procedure:

1. Develop a complete mathematical model consisting of all of the components of the Bubble CPAP system.
2. As there are two hypotheses on how Bubble CPAP helps in treating RDS (one based on the effect of pressure oscillation on the viscoelastic behavior of the lung and the other on the effect of pressure oscillations on surface tension dynamics), the lung model should incorporate both of these hypotheses. It should be able to:

    - Describe the viscoelastic and surface tension effects.
    - Produce the required assessment parameters as an output so that it can be compared to experiments. These parameters should be able to be measured in experiments and practice (preferably non-invasively).
    - Support clinical studies and identify mechanisms of improvement.

3. The common parameters used to study the respiratory system mechanics are compliance, resistance, impedance, and work of breath (WOB). Normally, these represent excellent displays of respiratory performance and their relationships to oxygen consumption make it possible to calculate the efficiency of the respiratory muscles. However, as they stand, they cannot describe the frequency dependence of the respiratory system and are either invasive procedures or require patient cooperation. Using the WOB

as an example, by measuring the relationship between the intrapleural pressure and lung volume, the work that has to be done to overcome the non-elastic and elastic forces in the respiratory system for a normal breath cycle can be determined. However, once pressure oscillations are added to the lung, the WOB graph no longer becomes useful. Thus it becomes difficult to analyze such a graph for any effect that the pressure oscillations may have on the WOB. Hence an alternative parameter is suggested and used which considers physiological performance in terms of the work of breath and pressure oscillation. This parameter is the power spectral density of the WOB.

1.4 MODELING PROCEDURE

There are several modeling concepts and procedures developed in the literature to analyze any physical or biological system; however, in this book we are limiting ourselves to the lumped parameter approach. For the type of systems we are dealing with in this book, this approach lends itself to simplicity, flexibility, and more relevance to the real systems at hand. The general approach is to follow these steps:

1. Define the system and its components.
2. Formulate a mathematical model.
3. Determine the system equations.
4. Solve for the desired output.
5. Validate the solution.
6. Analyze for design or performance.

Each system is broken down into several elements each of which can be analyzed and dealt with as a complete subsystem on its own. Coupling of each one of these elements must result in the complete original system in terms of characteristics and performance. Each one of these elements will be considered with only two ports to exchange energy with other elements of the system (Figure 1-2). The exchange of energy at each port requires the knowledge of two variables to define the energy at that port. In a general context, one of these variables is defined as the Flow variable (sometimes called the Through variable). An example of this variable is the charge in an electrical system, displacement in a mechanical system, and heat flow in a thermal system. The other variable is the Effort variable (sometimes called the Across variable). An example of this is the voltage in an electrical system, force in a mechanical system, and temperature in a thermal system.

Having defined the energy at each port, the energy flow through the element will be faced with some form of resistance. To avoid confusion with the standard definition of resistance and to generalize the concept, a

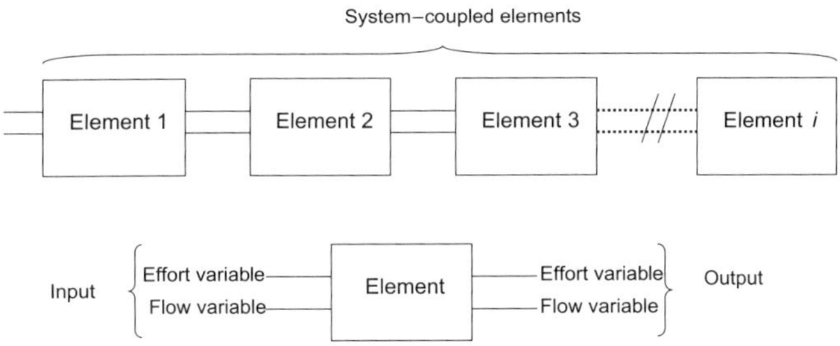

Figure 1-2. Two-port elements

more general definition is borrowed from electrical engineering, namely the impedance. As the impedance represents the net obstacle in a circuit, it combines resistances generated by resistors, inductors, and capacitors. Although these parameters are borrowed from electrical engineering, they have similar or equivalent parameters in all physical systems, including (but not limited to) mechanical, thermal, and fluid.

Once the element inputs and outputs are defined, the basic laws of physics are applied to determine the correlations between various element parameters and to achieve the objectives of the analysis. This may include determining the element or the system performance and/or characteristics. Although these physical laws, such as Newton's second law for force balance and Kirchhoff's law for voltage balance, may take different forms, they can all be formulated to follow a standard law of equilibrium. In principle, all of these laws can be formulated into a single law as follows:

$$\Sigma \textit{Potential difference across each element} = \textit{Net applied Effort Variable} \quad (1-1)$$

The potential difference across each element is defined as the product of the flow variable and the impedance. Equation (1-1) may be rewritten as:

$$\Sigma(\textit{Flow Variable} \times \textit{Impedance}) = \textit{Net applied Effort Variable} \quad (1-2)$$

The type of impedance changes in accordance with the nature of the element. Based on the nature of all physical systems treated in this book, electrical terminology may be borrowed to define three main types of impedances:

1. Resistive impedance
   If the resistance is defined by the symbol R, then the potential drop may be written as:

$$\textit{Resistive potential drop} = \textit{Flow Variable} \times R \qquad (1-3)$$

2. Inductive impedance
   If the inductance is defined by the symbol L, then the potential drop may be written as:

$$\textit{Inductive potential drop} = \textit{Flow Variable} \times LD \qquad (1-4)$$

   where D is the differential operator $D = \frac{d}{dt}$ and t is time.

3. Capacitive impedance
   If the capacitance is defined by the symbol C, then the potential drop may be written as:

$$\textit{Capacitive potential drop} = \textit{Flow Variable} \times 1/CD \qquad (1-5)$$

Equation (1-1) states a simple fact that the laws of nature have the same origin and can be summarized in a simple law of equilibrium. If the basic components of any system/element are known, the above equations can be used to analyze or investigate any system.

Consider the four basic systems dealt with in this book, electrical, mechanical, fluid and thermal systems. As indicated in Figure 1-3 all these systems share elements which have identical functions. Table 1-1 shows all these elements which can be summarized as follows:

1. Resistive Impedance: The resistive impedance is due to a resistance. The latter can be defined as the tendency of an element to oppose the flow (flow variable). This kind of impedance exists in electrical, mechanical, fluid and thermal systems.

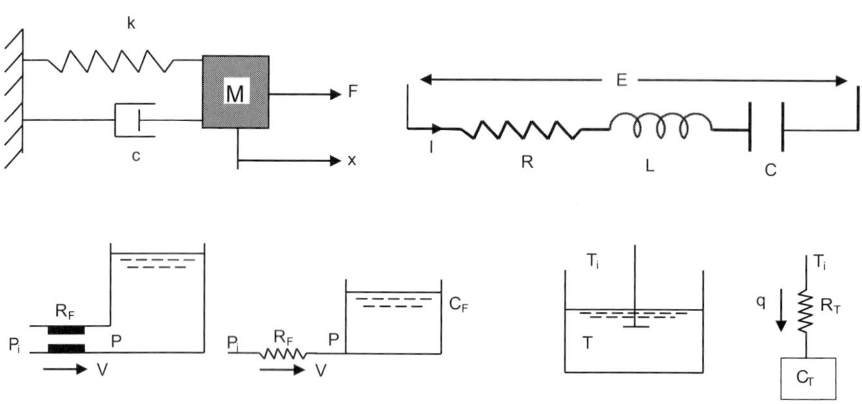

Figure 1-3. Four basic engineering systems and their elements

TABLE 1-1. Potential drops for various systems

System	Resistive	Capacitive	Inductive	Effort Variable	Flow Variable
Electrical	RDQ	Q/C	LD^2Q	Q	E
Mechanical	BDx	Kx	MD^2x	x	F
Fluid	R_FV	V/C_F	L_FDV	V	P
Thermal	R_Tq	q/C_T	Not defined	q	T

2. Capacitive Impedance: The capacitive impedance is due to the capacitance which is the storage of charge (flow variable). This kind of impedance exists in electrical, mechanical, fluid and thermal systems.
3. Inductive Impedance: The inductive impedance is due to the inductance in the system which results from the fact that a flow of current produces a magnetic field that tends to oppose the induced change in current. It is worth mentioning that inductance is defined in terms of inertia for an equivalent mechanical system and for a fluid system in terms of inertia effects encountered in accelerating a fluid in a pipe or passage. However, this is not defined for a thermal system.

Based on the above, Equation (1-1) can be written as follows:

1. For the electrical system with the charge Q as the flow variable and the voltage E as the effort variable, Equation (1-1) can be written as:

$$LD^2Q + RDQ + \frac{1}{C}Q = E \qquad (1-6)$$

where L, R, and C are the electrical inductance, resistance, and capacitance, respectively. The first, second, and third terms in this equation reflect the inductive, resistive, and capacitive potential drops, respectively.

2. For the mechanical system with the displacement x as the flow variable and the force F as the effort variable, Equation (1-1) can be written as:

$$MD^2x + BDx + Kx = F \qquad (1-7)$$

where M, B, and K are the mass, damping, and stiffness, respectively. The first, second and third terms in this equation reflect the inductive (inertial), resistive, and capacitive (storage) potential drop, respectively.

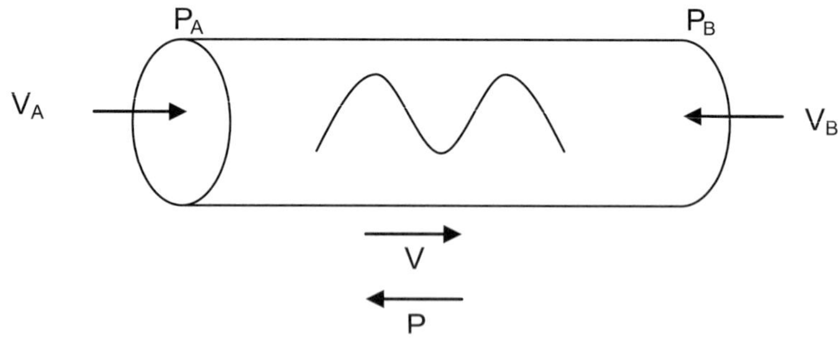

Figure 1-4. Elements of a fluid passage

3. Due to the nature of the fluid system, it might be difficult to write an equation similar to Equation (1-1); however, an alternative approach that deals with components rather than the complete system is presented here. The physical element called the pure fluid inductor represents the inertial effects encountered in accelerating a fluid in a pipe or passage (see Figure 1-4). An ideal fluid inductor is defined by the linear relation:

$$I(t) = L_f V(t) \quad (1-8)$$

and the pressure drop by:

$$P(t) = L_f DV(t) \quad (1-9)$$

where $I(t)$ is the inductor pressure momentum, $P(t)$ is the inductor pressure, $V(t)$ is the inductor volume flow; and the constant parameter $L_f\,[\mathrm{Pa.s^2m^{-3}}]$ is the fluid inductance or fluid inertance. However, for fluid resistance and capacitance, the following alternative formula can be used:

$$V = C_F DP = \frac{P_i - P}{R_F} \quad (1-10)$$

where the V is volume flow rate; P_i and P are the input and reservoir pressure, respectively; and R_F and C_F are the fluid resistance and capacitance, respectively.

4. Due to the nature of the thermal system, it is difficult to write an equation similar to Equation (1-1); however, an alternative approach similar to that of the fluid system by dealing with components rather than the complete system is dealt with. Also it is worth mentioning here that there is no definition for the thermal inductance and this will be disregarded here. For the thermal

resistance and capacitance, the following alternative formula can be used:

$$q = C_T DT = \frac{T_i - T}{R_T} \qquad (1-11)$$

where q is heat flow rate; T_i and T are the input and reservoir temperature, respectively; and R_T and C_T are the thermal resistance and capacitance, respectively.

Table 1-1 summarizes the potential drop defined in this context. With all these basic definitions, most of the elements in the following chapters can be modeled. However, some modifications are necessary depending on the situation.

To follow the "Talkative Model" approach given above, the equations in this section, or their derivatives, may be used to formulate two models: one for the device to be used for a particular treatment and another one for the physiological system for which the device will be used. Common assessment parameters have to be specified in order to determine how these parameters change when some physical parameters such as dimensions and materials within the device are modified.

1.5 CLOSURE

This chapter introduces the advantages of modeling and gives some simple modeling concepts as they are used for modeling lung therapy devices.

Part 1:

OBSTRUCTIVE SLEEP APNEA (OSA)

Chapter 2

OBSTRUCTIVE SLEEP APNEA: BASIC PRINCIPLES AND CURRENT TREATMENTS

This chapter provides a definition and overview of Obstructive Sleep Apnea (OSA), its pathophysiology, and diagnosis. Current treatments and devices that are part of the clinical management of OSA are also elaborated on, with particular attention to Continuous Positive Airway Pressure (CPAP) therapy.

2.1 OBSTRUCTIVE SLEEP APNEA (OSA)

OSA is defined by the presence of at least five obstructive events per hour during sleep in association with daytime sleepiness (somnolence). These obstructive events can be either brief periods of breathing cessation (apnea) or a marked reduction in tidal volume (hypopnea). According to these criteria, OSA occurs in 2% of women and 4% of men who are 30 to 60 years of age [1]. Risk factors for OSA include obesity, old age, systemic hypertension, increased neck circumference, craniofacial abnormalities, hypothyroidism, and acromegaly [2, 3]. Studies have associated OSA with an increased prevalence of cardiovascular and cerebrovascular disease, insulin resistance, and motor vehicle accidents. If untreated, OSA increases the risks of fatal and non-fatal cardiovascular events, which add billions of dollars to annual health-care costs [4-6].

The principal characteristic of OSA is the collapse of the upper airway during sleep. The site of the obstruction typically lies in the pharynx (see Figure 2-1). The muscles in the pharynx assist with swallowing and phonation. The dilating forces provided by the pharyngeal

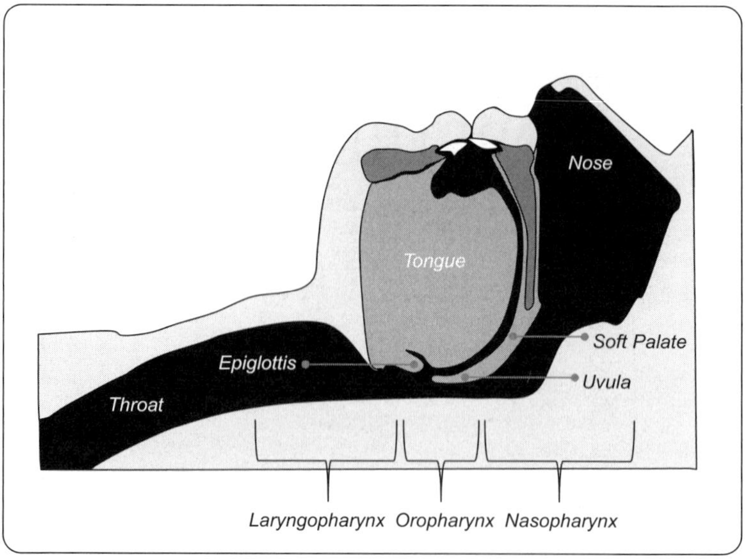

Figure 2-1. The pharynx: site of obstruction during OSA

muscles also provide pharyngeal patency during the breathing process [2, 5]. Factors that promote pharyngeal patency are increased transmural pressure, increased lung volume, and neck extension [7, 8]. Factors that narrow the pharyngeal airway are surface adhesive forces, neck flexion, jaw opening, and gravity [8, 9]. In healthy, awake subjects, the patency of the pharynx is maintained by continual neuromuscular activation of the pharyngeal muscles by the central nervous system. This activation is however reduced during sleep, which compromises the patency of the pharynx. This, in combination with abnormalities in airway structure, promotes the onset of OSA in varying degrees. Abnormalities of consequence include enlarged tonsils, uvula, and tongue; a low-hanging palate; and excess posterior pharyngeal tissue. The activation of dilator muscles in the pharynx is also reduced by alcohol, sleep deprivation, anesthesia, and sedative hypnotics [2, 5].

Complete obstruction of airflow (apnea) or partial obstruction (hypopnea) substantially reduces ventilation, which in turn results in hypercapnia and hypoxia. This stimulates arousal centers in the central nervous system to increase respiratory activity and triggers an arousal. Arousal restores the pharyngeal dilator muscle activity, thereby overcoming the obstruction, and ventilation resumes. Once the patient returns to sleep, the cycle repeats itself continuously throughout the night [10], as shown in Figure 2-2. The end of each cycle is associated with sleep fragmentation, peripheral vasoconstriction, as well as abrupt increases in systolic and diastolic blood pressures and heart rate [11].

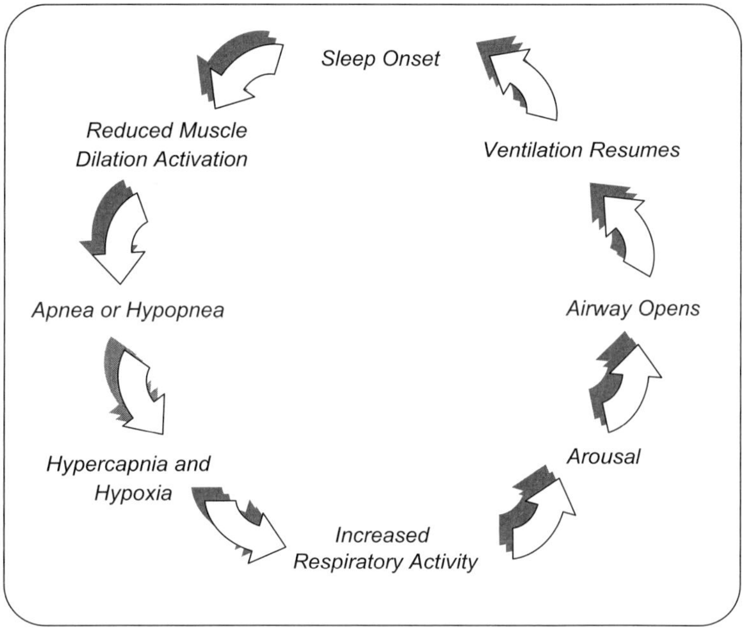

Figure 2-2. Pathophysiological sequence of typical OSA

2.2 DIAGNOSIS

OSA is diagnosed on the basis of clinical information and indices as well as laboratory testing. Physical examinations within the primary care setting identify patients with a high risk of OSA that meet the following criteria: disruptive snoring, daytime sleepiness, drowsiness while driving, obesity, and hypertension [12]. Other clinical variables such as neck circumference, body-mass index (BMI), and other craniofacial and soft tissue conditions that increase upper airway resistance are also used to predict OSA [3, 13].

Polysomnography is the recommended diagnostic test for OSA and other sleep-related breathing disorders [14, 15]. A patient undergoing a polysomnogram is shown in Figure 2-3. The standard polysomnogram is a combination of the following laboratory-based recordings [3, 13–15]:

- Electroencephalography (EEG) – recordings of electrical activity along the scalp by electrodes to detect arousal from sleep.
- Electrooculography (EOG) – recordings of eye movement by electrodes placed either on or around the eye.

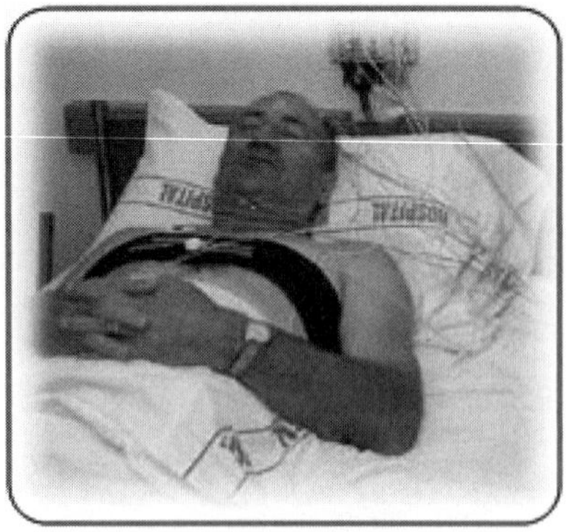

Figure 2-3. A patient undergoing a polysomnogram [Reproduced with permission from Fisher & Paykel Healthcare Ltd]

- Electromyography (EMG) – recordings of muscle movement with electrodes on the chest, abdomen, and mouth to record respiratory movements, and additional electrodes on the limbs to record limb movements.
- Electrocardiography (ECG) – recordings of the electrical activity of the heart with skin electrodes.
- Nasal and oral airflow and pressure – to measure respiratory activity.
- Oximetry – to measure the oxygenation of the blood with a pulse oximeter.

2.3 CLINICAL MANAGEMENT AND TREATMENT OF OSA

2.3.1 Oral Devices

Oral devices are appropriate for subjects who do not respond to, or are not candidates for, treatments that involve lifestyle modifications such as weight loss or sleep-position change. Although not as efficacious in the treatment of OSA as CPAP therapies (discussed in section 2.3.3), oral devices are also recommended for patients with mild to moderate OSA who prefer these devices to CPAP therapies or who do not respond to CPAP. These devices are therefore used mainly by patients who snore but have only mild apnea [14, 16]. Oral devices can be divided into two main groups [5, 16–18]: those that move the mandible forward and those that move the tongue forward, thus increasing the airway space in the posterior pharyngeal area. These are briefly described as follows:

- Mandibular repositioning devices [19] (Figure 2-4) – These fit tightly over the patient's teeth and pull the bottom jaw forward. They are suitable for patients with normal- size tongues and soft palates.
- Tongue retaining devices [20] (Figure 2-5) – These are soft polyvinyl devices that fit over the patient's teeth or gums. An anterior bulb that projects beyond the lips holds the tongue in place by means of negative pressure created by the displacement of air in the bubble by the tongue. These are suitable for patients with large tongues, no teeth, or who cannot advance their mandible.

2.3.2 Surgical Treatment

Those patients who cannot be treated adequately with conservative, non-invasive measures or who have significant craniofacial abnormalities are more effectively treated with the following surgical procedures [5, 13, 16]. Uvulopalatoplasty is a surgical or laser procedure that removes part of the uvula and soft palate. Radiofrequency techniques can also be used to reduce the size of the palatal soft tissue. Such palatal procedures, however, show subjective improvements in snoring and are not consistently effective in treating sleep apnea since many patients have airway obstructions beyond the palatal areas that cannot be treated by soft tissue procedures.

For patients who cannot be treated by soft palate surgery, maxillomandibular advancement surgery can be considered to effectively treat OSA. Adolescents and young adults who cannot tolerate non-invasive treatments

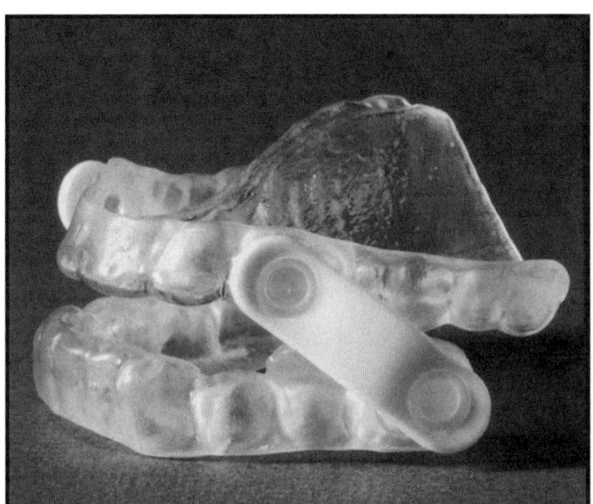

Figure 2-4. Mandibular repositioning device [Courtesy of Henke et al. [19]]

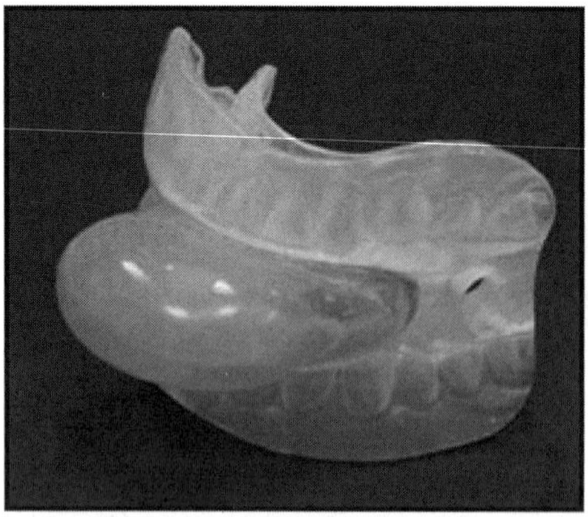

Figure 2-5. Tongue retaining device [Courtesy of Lazard et al. [20]]

and are healthy enough to undergo extensive surgery may also be candidates for maxillomandibular advancement procedures. However, complications include bleeding, infections, hematoma, and facial anesthesia and so patients need close postoperative monitoring in intensive care units.

If all other treatment options fail, a tracheostomy can be considered as a last-resort measure, especially for morbidly obese patients with severe OSA and patients with acute respiratory failure. This is not a well-accepted long-term treatment, however, due to the associated complications and disability resulting from such a procedure.

2.3.3 CPAP Therapy

Nasal CPAP as a treatment for OSA was first reported in 1981. Since then, it has been regarded as the most consistent and effective treatment for OSA, and is widely used because of its ease of application [2, 13, 16, 21]. It provides air at positive pressure through a nasal or facial mask, creating a pneumatic splint that keeps the pharyngeal airway open during inspiration and expiration (see Figure 2-6). Typical CPAP systems, as shown in Figure 2-7, consist of a fan that blows air under low pressure (which can typically vary between 3 to 20 cm H_2O) into the patient interface through a flexible hose. To combat nasal dryness and irritation, cool or heated humidification is often added between the fan and the mask. This increases patient compliance and device use by preventing drying of the mucous membranes of the upper airway [16, 22, 23].

The level of air pressure required for CPAP therapy is titrated during polysomnography, often during the same night as the diagnostic study. The titration pressure is identified as the minimum pressure at which obstructive events are prevented, thus maintaining normal levels of oxygenation and decreasing the frequency of arousals from sleep

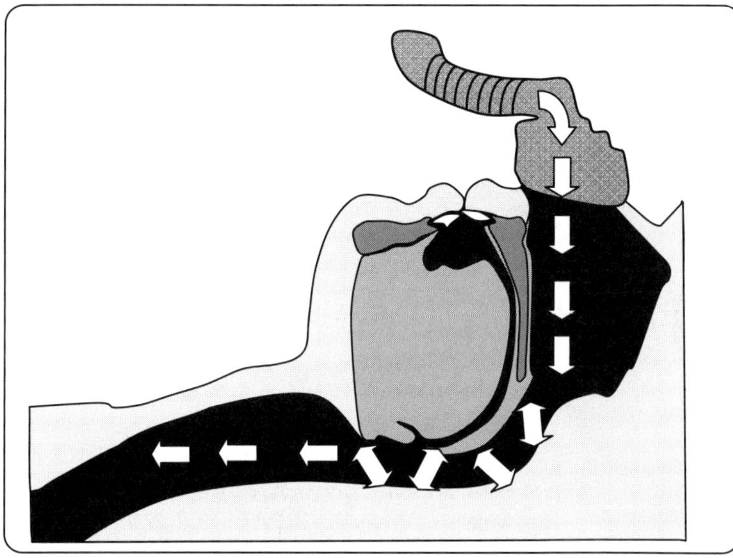

Figure 2-6. CPAP treatment providing a pneumatic splint in the pharynx

[5, 14, 24]. CPAP requirements may change over time with weight loss, weight gain, or age, and CPAP pressures may need to be reassessed if symptoms return [16].

The optimal interface is also ideally determined during polysomnography. A wide variety of interfaces, which range from full-face masks to nasal interfaces (a mask or a pillow system), are available in a variety of sizes, shapes, and materials to maximize patient comfort (see Figure 2-8). Full-face masks are used for preferential mouth breathers or in cases where air leakage from the mouth cannot be controlled. Chin straps, head gear, and gel and cushioning interfaces are also available to improve compliance and prevent abrasions and skin breakdown [2, 5, 13, 16].

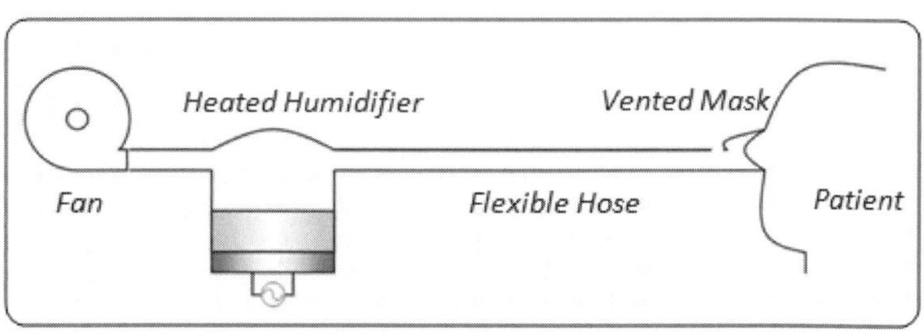

Figure 2-7. Components of a typical CPAP system

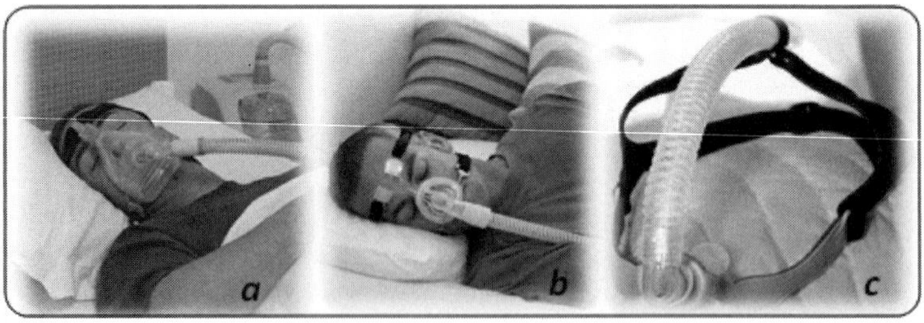

Figure 2-8. CPAP interfaces: (a) full-face mask, (b) nasal mask and (c) nasal pillow [Reproduced with permission from Fisher & Paykel Healthcare Ltd]

Although fixed pressure CPAP is effective in most patients, other modes of pressure delivery can be considered, such as Bi-level Positive Airway Pressure (BiPAP) and auto-Adjusting (or Autotitrating) Positive Airway Pressure (APAP). These techniques are intended to improve patient comfort and compliance, and if tolerated may prove useful in selected patients. However, there is no convincing evidence in the literature that any of these modified forms of CPAP have better compliance or efficacy than fixed-pressure CPAP, and so additional research is necessary before their use is widely recommended [2, 5, 25–27].

BiPAP is an optional treatment that can be used where the patient experiences difficulty or discomfort when exhaling against a fixed pressure [28]. Pressure is maintained through a pressure-controlled valve at two different preset higher and lower levels during inspiration and expiration, respectively. The Inspiratory Positive Airway Pressure (IPAP) is equivalent to the pressure of conventional mechanical ventilation techniques and the Expiratory Positive Airway Pressure (EPAP) is equivalent to the external end-positive airway pressure [25, 29]. Such a technique seeks to relieve OSA at lower expiratory pressures than during conventional CPAP therapy, thereby reducing the potential for barotrauma, mechanical ventilatory depression, and reduction of cardiac output associated with high mean airway pressures [30]. APAP was developed in the last decade with the intention of continuously adjusting pressure to meet the variable needs of a patient. The pressure is adjusted based on feedback from various respiratory measures such as snoring (airway vibration), airflow (apnea or hypopnea), and the flow versus time profile (airflow limitation) and respiratory impedance via the forced oscillation technique. Some units utilize a built-in pneumotachograph to quantify flow and the flow versus time profile, while other machines use differences in blower speed during inspiration and exhalation. Most APAP devices start with a baseline pressure (usually around 3 to 4 cm H_2O) and then titrate upward as needed. An absence of monitored events then prompts a gradual decrease in pressure. This allows the minimum effective pressure to be delivered in a given circumstance. The APAP devices usually allow the clinician to set maximum and minimum pressure limits [31, 32].

2.4 CLOSURE

This chapter has covered the pathophysiology of OSA along with current practices in its diagnoses and treatment. Particular attention is drawn to Nasal CPAP therapy since it is the most widely used and effective treatment for OSA.

REFERENCES

[1] Young, T., Palta, M., Dempsey, J., Skatrud, J., Weber, S., Badr, S., 1993, The occurrence of sleep disordered breathing among middle aged adults, *N Engl J Med*, **328**, p. 1230–1235.

[2] Basner, R.C., 2007, Continuous Positive Airway Pressure for Obstructive Sleep Apnea, *N Engl J Med*, **356**, p. 1751–1758.

[3] Flemons, W.W., 2002, Obstructive Sleep Apnea. *N Engl J Med*, **347**(7), p. 498–504.

[4] Punjabi, N.M., et al., 2004, Sleep disordered breathing, glucose intolerance and insulin resistance: The Sleep Heart Health Study, *Am J Epidemiol*, **160**, p. 521–530.

[5] Qureshi, A. and Ballard, R.D., 2003, Obstructive Sleep Apnea, *J Allergy Clin Immunol*, **112**, p. 643–651.

[6] Shahar, E., et al., 2001, Sleep-disordered breathing and cardiovascular disease: cross-sectional results of the Sleep Heart Health Study, *Am J Respir Crit Care Med*, **163**, p. 19–25.

[7] Hoffstein, V., Zamel, N., and Phillipson, E.A., 1984, Lung volume dependence of pharyngeal cross-sectional area in patients with obstructive sleep apnea, *Am Rev Respir Dis*, **130**, p. 175–8.

[8] Morikawa, S., Safar, P., and DeCarlo, J., 1981, Influence of the head-jaw position upon upper airway patency. *Anesthesiology*, **22**, p. 265–70.

[9] Koenig, J.S. and Thach, B.T., 1988, Effect of mass loading on the upper airway, *J Appl Physiol*, **64**, p. 2124–2131.

[10] Gleeson, K., Zwillich, C.W., and White, D.P., 1990, The influence of increasing ventilatory effort on arousal from sleep, *Am Rev Respir Dis*, **142**, p. 295–300.

[11] Garpestad, E., Katayama, H., Parker, J.A., Ringler, J., Lilly, J., Yasuda, T., Moore, R.H., Strauss, H.W., Weiss, J.W., 1992, Stroke volume and cardiac output decrease at termination of obstructive apneas, *J Appl Physiol*, **73**, p. 1743–1748.

[12] Netzer, N.C., Stoohs, R.A., Netzer, C.M., Clark, K., Strohl, K.P., 1999, Using the Berlin Questionnaire to identify patients at risk for the sleep apnea syndrome, *Ann Intern Med*, **131**, p. 485–491.

[13] Olson, E.J., Moore, W.R., Morgenthaler, T., Gay, P.C., Staats, B.A., 2003, Obstructive Sleep Apnea-Hypopnea Syndrome, *Mayo Clinic Proceedings*, **78**(12), p. 1545–1552.

[14] Kushida, C.A., Littner, M.R., Morgenthaler, T., Alessi, C.A., Bailey, D., Coleman, J., Friedman, L., Hirshkowitz, M., Kapen, S., Kramer, M., Lee-Chiong, T., Loube,

D.L., Owens, J., Pancer, J.P., Wise, M., 2005, Practice parameters for the indications for polysomnography and related procedures: an update for 2005, *Sleep*, **28**(4), p. 499–521.

[15] Polysomnography Task Force and American Sleep Disorders Association Standards of Practice Committee, 1997, Practice parameters for the indications for polysomnography and related procedures, *Sleep*, **20**, p. 406–422.

[16] Victor, L.D., 2004, Treatment of Obstructive Sleep Apnea in Primary Care, *American Family Physician*, **69**(3), p. 561–568.

[17] Saletu, A., Anderer, P., Parapatics, S., Matthai, C., Matejka, M., Saletu, B., 2007, Effects of a Mandibular Repositioning Appliance on Sleep Structure, Morning Behavior and Clinical Symptomatology in Patients with Snoring and Sleep-Disordered Breathing, *Neuropsychobiology*, **55**, p. 184–193.

[18] Lowe, A.A., 1999, Titratable Oral Appliances for the Treatment of Snoring and Obstructive Sleep Apnea, *J Can Dent Assoc*, **65**, p. 571–574.

[19] Henke, K.G., Frantz, D.E., and Kuna, S.T., 2000, An Oral Elastic Mandibular Advancement Device for Obstructive Sleep Apnea, *Am J Respir Crit Care Med*, **161**(2), p. 420–425.

[20] Lazard, D.S., Blumen, M., Lévy, P., Chauvin, P., Fragny, D., Buchet, I., Chabolle, F., 2009, The Tongue-Retaining Device: Efficacy and Side Effects in Obstructive Sleep Apnea Syndrome, *J Clin Sleep Med*, **5**(5), p. 431–438.

[21] Sullivan, C.E., et al., 1981, Reversal of obstructive sleep apnea by continuous positive airway pressure applied through the nares, *Lancet*, **1**, p. 862–865.

[22] Rakotonanahary, D., et al., 2001, Predictive factors for the need for additional humidification during nasal continuous positive airway pressure therapy, *Chest*, **119**, p. 460–465.

[23] Massie, C.A., Hart, R.W., Peralez, K., Richards, G.N., 1999, Effects of humidification on nasal symptoms and compliance in sleep apnea patients using continuous positive airway pressure, *Chest*, **116**, p. 403–408.

[24] Loube, D.I., Gay, P.C., Strohl, K.P., Pack, A.I., White, D.P., Collop, N.A., 1999, Indications for positive airway pressure treatment of adult obstructive sleep apnea patients: a consensus statement, *Chest*, **115**, p. 863–866.

[25] Chan, C.K., et al., 1998, Bilevel positive airway pressure nasal mask ventilation in patients with acute hypercapnic respiratory failure, *Hong Kong Medical Journal*, **4**(2), p. 125–131.

[26] Reeves-Hoché, M.K., et al., 1995, Continuous versus bilevel positive airway pressure for obstructive sleep apnea, *Am J Respir Crit Care Med*, **151**, p. 443–449.

[27] Ayas, N.T., et al., 2004, Auto-titrating versus standard continuous positive airway pressure for the treatment of obstructive sleep apnea: results of a meta-analysis, *Sleep*, **27**, p. 249–253.

[28] Kushida, C.A., Littner, M.R., Hirshkowitz, M., Morgenthaler, T.I., Alessi, C.A., Bailey, D., Boehlecke, B., Brown, T.M., Coleman, J., Friedman, L., Kapen, S., Kapur, V.K., Kramer, M., Lee-Chiong, T., Owens, J., Pancer, J.P., Swick, T.J., Wise, M.S., 2006, Practice Parameters for the Use of Continuous and Bilevel Positive Airway Pressure Devices to Treat Adult Patients With Sleep-Related Breathing Disorders, *Sleep*, **29**(3), p. 375–380.

[29] Braghiroli, A. and Donner, C.F., 1992, Bilevel positive airway pressure, *Eur Respir Rev*, **2**, p. 398–399.

[30] Sanders, M.H. and Kern, N., 1990, Obstructive sleep apnea treated by independently adjusted inspiratory and expiratory positive airway pressures via nasal mask: physiologic and clinical implications, *Chest*, **98**(2), p. p317(8).

[31] Berry, R.B., Parish, J.M., and Hartse, K.M., 2002, The Use of Auto-Titrating Continuous Positive Airway Pressure for Treatment of Adult Obstructive Sleep Apnea, *Sleep*, **25**(2), p. 148–173.

[32] Morgenthaler, T.I., Aurora, R.,N., Brown, T., Zak, R., Alessi, C., Boehlecke, B., Chesson Jr, A.L., Friedman, L., Kapur, V., Maganti, R., Owens, J., Pancer, J., Swick, T.J., 2008, Practice Parameters for the Use of Autotitrating Continuous Positive Airway Pressure Devices for Titrating Pressures and Treating Adult Patients with Obstructive Sleep Apnea Syndrome: An Update for 2007, **31**(1), p. 141–147.

Chapter 3

MODELING OF CONTINUOUS POSITIVE AIRWAY PRESSURE (CPAP)

In this chapter a lumped parameter approach for modeling a typical air breather such as the Continuous Positive Airway Pressure (CPAP) device is presented. It is assumed that the reader is familiar with the basic laws of physics and engineering curricula that are applied to generate models that are implemented in Simulink™ in the Matlab™ environment. It is important to acknowledge that the primary aim of such models is to help the engineering design process. The challenge therein lies in the ability of the model to incorporate as many design parameters as are necessary to adequately describe the dynamic behavior of the system for the purposes required, while reducing model complexity by sacrificing details that have insignificant effects on system dynamics. The manner in which model components as well as the overall model can be validated experimentally is shown here.

The objective of modeling techniques in this book is to produce practical models based on realistic assumptions, as opposed to hypothetical models based on highly idealized assumptions. Such models (as presented in this chapter) could be used for one of many objectives, including optimization, determination of various design parameters, development of new components, or as a good educational exercise of the modeling process undertaken in lung supportive devices. The example presented at the end of this chapter models a prototype CPAP device in order to test its performance when particular design parameters are changed.

3.1 PRINCIPLES OF OPERATION AND SYSTEM COMPONENTS

Figure 3-1 shows a typical breather that consists of four main components: Air Delivery Unit (ADU), a humidification unit, a heated tube,

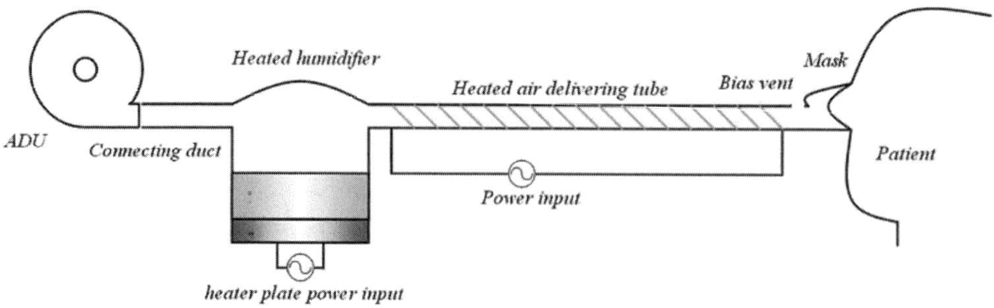

Figure 3-1. Typical breather components

and a mask. The air delivery unit consists of an air compressor, a delivery duct, and a control unit. It provides and maintains a proper positive pressure to the mask and then to the patient's airway. The connecting duct guides the airflow into the humidifier chamber. The humidification unit consists of a heater, a humidification chamber, and a temperature controller. The heated delivery tube consists of a corrugated tube with a heating coil. As the tube wall temperature is lower than the supplied humidifier air temperature, it is essential to heat the tube in order to avoid condensation. In practice, the pressure in the mask is usually kept within 0.05 kPa. The mask is the main interface with the patient and it has several bias flow holes to pass the exhaled air out of the mask and to expel carbon dioxide. This chapter presents a simplified model of the system that focuses on fluid modeling and reserves the thermodynamic considerations of the system (associated with the humidification process) to Chapter 4.

3.2 LUMPED PARAMETER MODELING OF COMPONENTS

Figure 3-2 shows the various components of a typical CPAP system. To develop an overall system model, each one of these components must be analyzed to produce unit models, which are then combined to give the system model. These models are obtained by incorporating the fluid and element characteristics such flow resistances, inertance, physical properties, flexible air delivery tube compliance, and mask compliance into the state, continuity, and momentum equations.

As a simplified but realistic model is sought, the following assumptions are made:

1. The thermodynamic gas processes are assumed to be isothermal, since changes in pressure are sufficiently low and the system operates at room temperature.
2. The effect of mass transfer from water contained within the humidification reservoir is ignored.

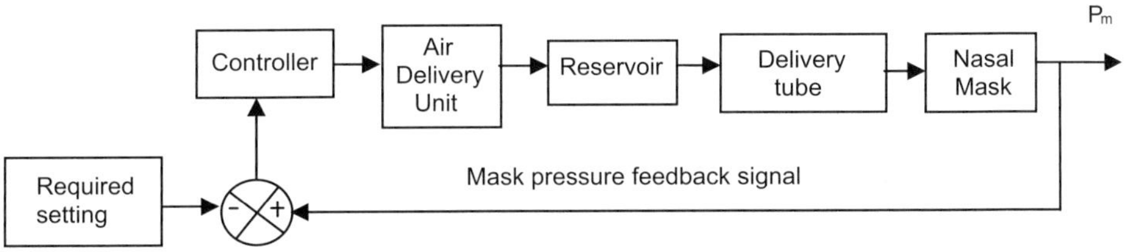

Figure 3-2. Block diagram of the CPAP system model showing physical parameters considered

3. The effects of non-linear system characteristics, such as turbulent flow resistance and orifice discharge characteristics, are linearized over the system's normal operation range. Linearization is a commonly used approximation technique to convert non-linear models into more tractable linear ones.

In the following sections, the derivation of each model block is developed, and then assembled to form the completed system model. There is usually a specific purpose for developing any model. This could be for design optimization, assessment of system performance, or any other development or research objectives. At the end of the chapter the model is experimentally validated as well as applied to assess the performance of a system under parametric variations.

3.2.1 Air Delivery Unit

The main element of the air delivery unit is the compressor. This could be reciprocating, rotary, diaphragm, or any other type of suitable compressor. However, the most common type is the centrifugal compressor (rotary type). See Appendix A for more details. As the main purpose of the compressor is to deliver the required air pressure and flow rates, it is assumed that the compressor is a zero type system with an output directly proportional to the input at this stage.

3.2.2 Connecting Duct

This kind of duct is normally built with rigid walls within the compressor housing. As the wall is rigid, the flow through the duct is modeled as a purely resistive element. Any accumulation effects due to the compressibility of air are neglected. Further, the dependence of the pressure drop on the mass flow rate through the duct is also neglected. The design flow rate is used to determine the "mean flow resistance" of the tube. Figure 3-3 illustrates the pressures at each end of the tube and flow rate through it. The mass flow rate $\dot{m}_d$ through the connecting duct is given by:

$$\dot{m}_d = \frac{P_d - P_r}{R_d} \qquad (3-1)$$

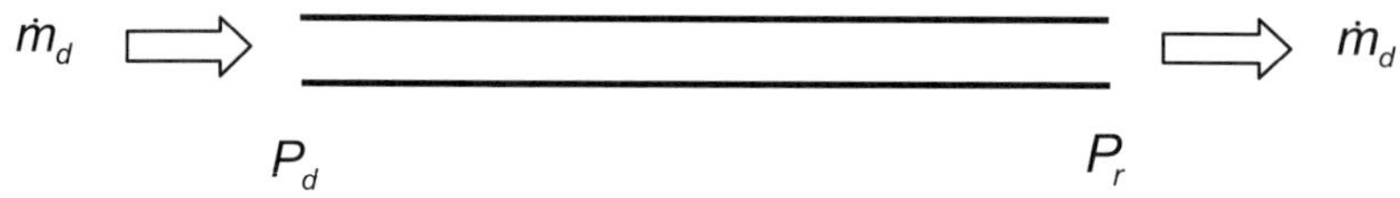

Figure 3-3. Modeling of the discharge tube

where R_d is the mean flow resistance of the connecting duct; and P_d and P_r are the connecting duct and reservoir pressures, respectively.

3.2.3 Reservoir

Assumptions and Simplifications: Humidification is a necessary process in most lung therapy devices. Dry air causes airway dryness, irritation, and patient discomfort. This process is normally achieved by using various humidification techniques. The reservoir may represent this process. In this section changes in air properties are neglected, since it is assumed that the process is isothermal due to the very low pressure variation experienced.

Derivation: The pressure inside the reservoir depends on the mass of air held within the reservoir (Figure 3-4), which is determined by the inflow and outflow rates and the accumulation rate of air. Over a period of time *dt,* the continuity equation (mass in-mass out= mass storage) over the reservoir, can be written as:

$$(\dot{m}_c - \dot{m}_s)dt = dM_r \qquad (3-2)$$

where $\dot{m}_c$ and $\dot{m}_s$ are the air mass flow rate delivered to and supplied by the humidification reservoir, respectively; and M_r is the total mass of air within the reservoir. The mass of air in the reservoir can be related to the pressure using the equation of state. If we assume that there is no change in temperature, the equation of state for the air mass in the reservoir is given by:

$$P_r V_r = M_r R_a T_r \qquad (3-3)$$

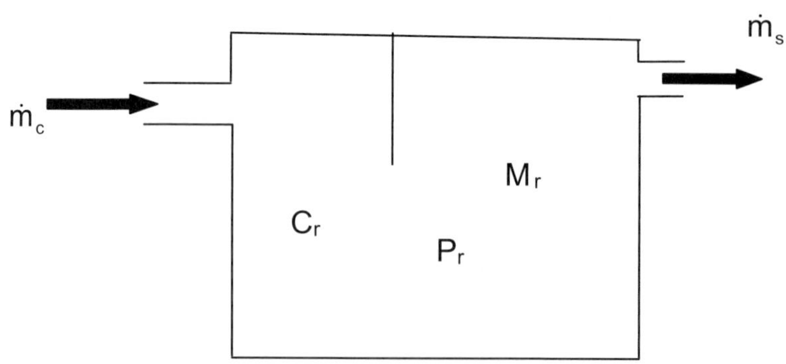

Figure 3-4. Schematic representation of the reservoir

where V_r and T_r are volume and temperature of the air mass in the reservoir; and R_a is the gas constant for air. Assuming constant temperature and volume results in:

$$\frac{dM_r}{dt} = \frac{V_r}{R_a T_r}\frac{dP_r}{dt} \qquad (3-4)$$

Using this equation, equation (3-2) can be rewritten as:

$$\dot{m}_c - \dot{m}_s = C_r \frac{dP_r}{dt} \qquad (3-5)$$

where the reservoir capacitance $C_r = V_r/R_a T_r$.

3.2.4 Delivery Tube

Assumptions and Simplifications: In most modeling cases the behavior of this type of tube may be assumed as purely resistive; however, due to the relatively high peak air velocity within the delivery tube, it is necessary to consider both the air inertia and shear flow resistance. To simplify the tube analysis, the following assumptions are made:

1. Both the air and flexible tube wall are combined to determine an equivalent effective bulk modulus.
2. Due to the relatively low peak pressures involved, the compliance effect can be neglected without any significant effect on the dynamic behavior of the model. The fluctuating patient breathing load experienced by the model (Figure 3-5) ranges from 0.7 g/s outflow to 0.3 g/s inflow, during inhalation and expiration, respectively, and is based on an average adult patient breathing at rest [1].

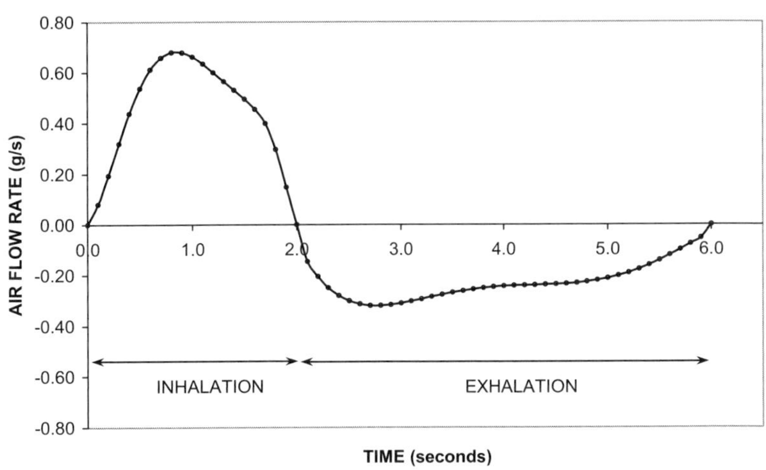

Figure 3-5. Breathing cycle at rest (Measured Data)

To achieve a constant mask pressure, typical commercially available breathing systems that deal with fluctuating breathing loads require the mask air mass inflow rate to range from 1.4 g/s down to 0.7 g/s during patient inhalation and exhalation, respectively. Nasal mask air pressures of 16 cm H_2O typically produce a continuous mask vent bias flow of 0.7 g/s. The average diameter of a delivery tube is about 5 cm. Thus, during patient breathing, the air velocity within the tube ranges from 15 m/s up to 45.3 m/s, based on the fluctuating mask air mass inflow rate. The maximum rate of acceleration of the tube airflow is in the order of 30.3 m/s^2, requiring the resulting inertia effect to be considered.

Derivation: Figure 3-6 shows a control volume surrounding the air within the tube. The main forces to be considered are caused by the pressure from both sides of the tube and friction. Applying Newton's second law across the control volume results in:

$$(K_s P_r - P_m)A_t - P_f A_t = -\rho_a A_t L_t \frac{dV_t}{dt} \qquad (3-6)$$

where K_s is the reservoir contraction shock loss; P_r and P_m are the reservoir and mask pressure, respectively; A_t is the tube cross-sectional area; P_f is the air shear resistance force; ρ_a is the air density; L_t is the tube length; and V_t is the air velocity within the tube.

The pressure drop along the delivery tube is mainly due to wall shear forces and it represents the single most significant impact on both the pressure attenuation and dynamic behavior of the breathing system. This can be determined using the following equation:

$$P_{f_t} = \frac{f L_t \dot{m}_t^2}{2d_t - \rho_a A_t^2} \qquad (3-7)$$

where L_t, d_t, A_t and $\dot{m}_t$ are the tube length, diameter, area, and mass flow rate, respectively. The friction coefficient f can be determined after knowing the flow regime under consideration. For the average tube dimensions given above, the minimum Reynolds number is about 2800 for a minimum airflow of 0.4 g/s. The tube inner wall is corrugated as seen in Figure 3-7. However, since the relative roughness is small, the pitch is long, and the Reynolds number is no more than 105, the inner surface

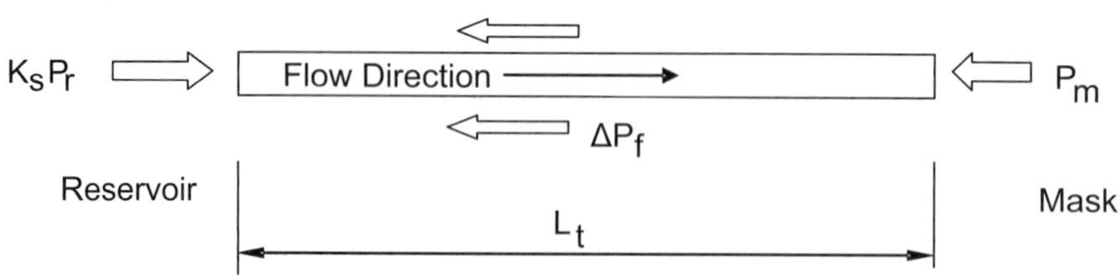

Figure 3-6. Air delivery tube control volume

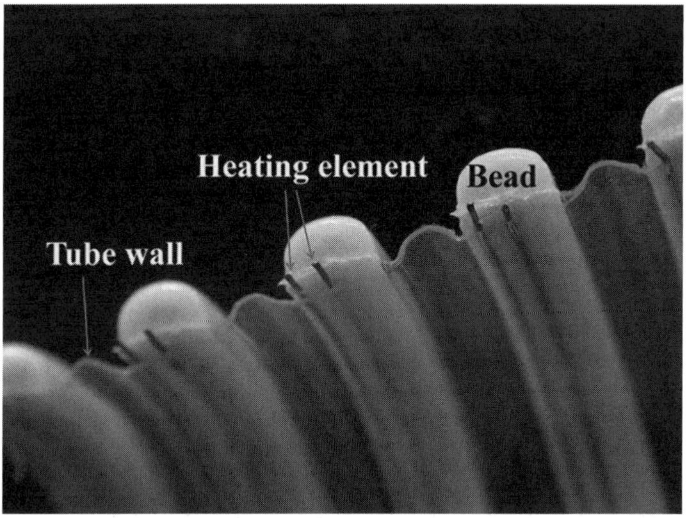

Figure 3-7. Corrugated wall delivery tube [Courtesy of F&P Healthcare Ltd]

friction may not be significantly different from that of a smooth tube. The following Darcy-Weisbach friction factor can be used [2]:

$$f = \frac{0.3164}{\mathrm{Re}^{0.25}} \qquad (3-8)$$

If we assume no mass storage within the tube, then the tube mass flow rate $\dot{m}_t = \dot{m}_s$. The air velocity within the tube may be written as:

$$V_t = \dot{m}_t / \rho_a A_t \qquad (3-9)$$

Substituting this into equation (3-7) gives the pressure drop along the tube.

An experimental investigation was conducted to determine the accuracy of equation (3-7). Figure 3-8 indicates that both the experimental and predicted values are in excellent agreement. A typical tube, where the air mass inflow rate varies between 1.4 and 0.6 g/s to achieve a constant nasal mask pressure of 16 cm H_2O, requires a mean operating value of 1 g/s to be used for linearization purposes. Using the slope at this point results in a straight line that is slightly offset to minimize any error over the breathing system operating range. This method of approximation is quite accurate as long as normal operation is not too far from the operating point. The percentage error present between the predicted linear and non-linear values, over the calculated system air mass flow range, varies from +4% to –11% [1]. Thus the linearizd model for the friction within the tube may be determined in terms of the slope (R_m) and the intercept (Y_m) as:

$$\Delta P_f = R_m \dot{m}_t + Y_m \qquad (3-10)$$

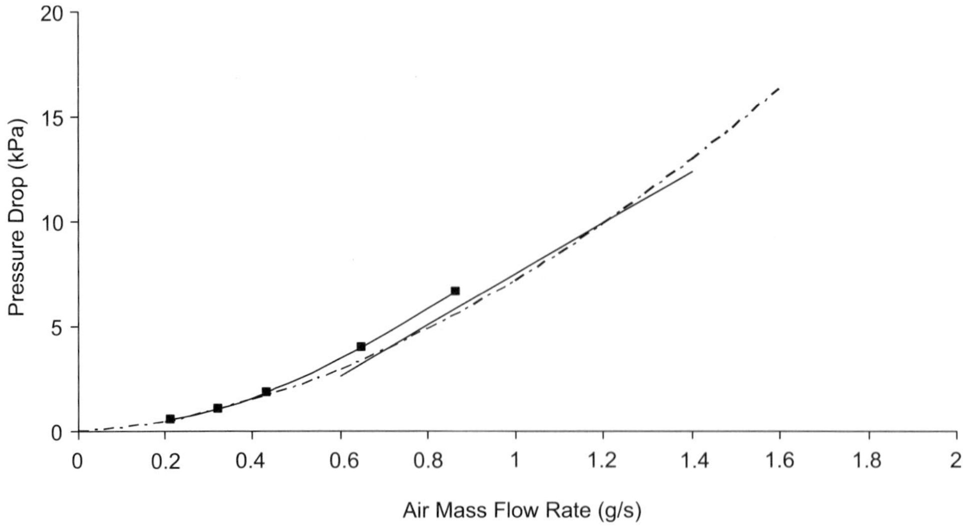

Figure 3-8. Pressure drop along a 5.5mm internal diameter PVC tube; measured, predicted, — linear model [1]

where the subscript m refers to tube air mass flow in the $\Delta P_f - \dot{m}_t$ curve. This pressure drop may also be represented in terms of the pressure difference experienced at either end as:

$$\Delta P_f = K_s P_r - P_m \tag{3-11}$$

Combining equations (3-10) and (3-11) gives the air mass flow rate within the tube expressed in terms of the linearized resistance and air pressure experienced at either end of the tube, namely:

$$\dot{m}_t = \frac{(K_s P_r - P_m - Y_m)}{R_m} \tag{3-12}$$

Substituting this into equation (3 – 5) leads to:

$$\dot{m}_c - \frac{(K_s P_r - P_m - Y_m)}{R_m} = C_r \frac{dP_r}{dt} \tag{3-13}$$

Introducing the D-operator, where $D = \dfrac{d}{dt_m}$ and rearranging equation (3-13) yields the following expression for the breathing system reservoir pressure (P_r):

$$\frac{P_r}{\dot{m}_c + \dfrac{P_m}{R_m} + \dfrac{Y_m}{R_m}} = \frac{\dfrac{R_m}{K_s}}{\dfrac{R_m}{K_s}(C_r D + 1)} \tag{3-14}$$

Combining equation (3-10) with equation (3-6) leads to:

$$K_s P_r - P_m - (R_m + Y_m) = \rho_a L_t D V_t \qquad (3-15)$$

Rearranging equation (3-15) yields an expression for tube air velocity (V_t) as:

$$\frac{V_t}{K_s P_r - P_m - Y_m} = \frac{\frac{1}{R_m}}{\frac{\rho_a L_t}{R_m} D + 1} \qquad (3-16)$$

3.2.5 Mask

Assumptions and Simplifications: Air is supplied to the patient via a mask that is continually purged through small vents, ensuring that fresh air is always available to breathe. Typical masks are shown in Figure 3-9. Again, due to the very low pressure variation, changes in air properties are neglected since it is assumed that the process is isothermal. The mask may be considered as another reservoir as shown in Figure 3-10. In a period of *dt, a*pplying the mass continuity equation leads to:

$$(\dot{m}_t - \dot{m}_b \pm \dot{m}_p)dt = dm_m \qquad (3-17)$$

where $\dot{m}_t$, $\dot{m}_b$, and $\dot{m}_p$ are the air mass flow rates entering from the tube, and exiting from the mask vents (called bias flow) and from the fluctuating patient

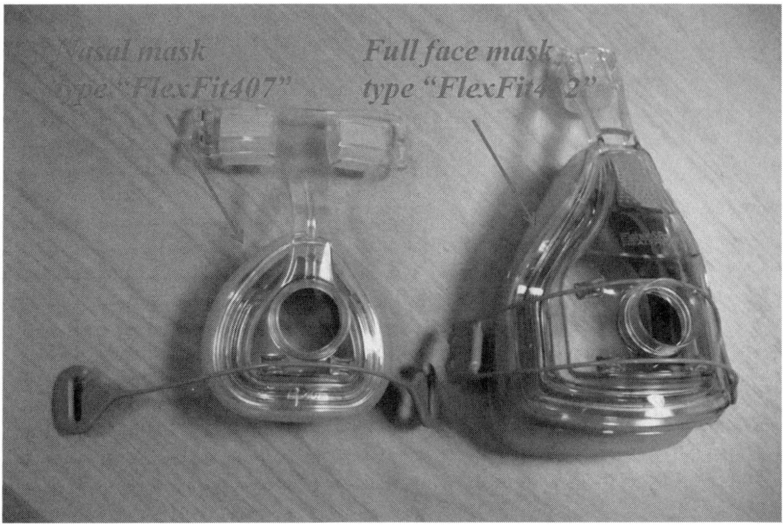

Figure 3-9. Typical masks [Courtesy of Fisher & Paykel Healthcare Ltd]

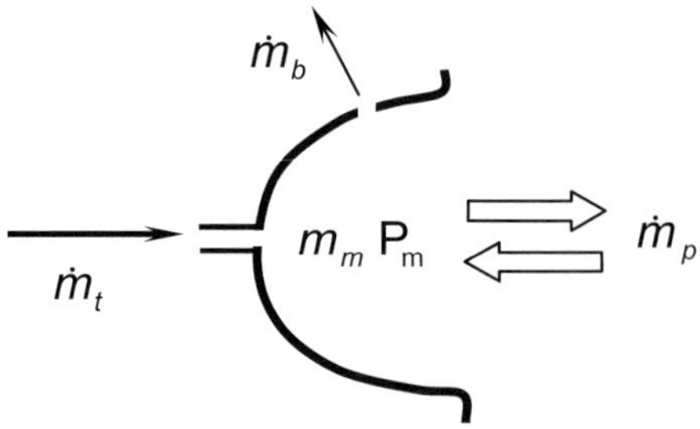

Figure 3-10. Schematic representation of a mask model

breathing, respectively; m_m is the total mass of air contained within mask; and the "±" reflects the inhalation and exhalation process, respectively.

To determine the rate of change of air mass contained within the mask, the following equation of state is used:

$$P_m V_m = m_m R_a T_m \tag{3-18}$$

where P_m, V_m, and T_m are the mask pressure, volume, and temperature, respectively. Assuming constant temperature and volume results in:

$$\frac{dm_m}{dt} = \frac{dP_m}{dt}\frac{V_m}{R_a T_m} \tag{3-19}$$

Substituting this into equation (3-17) results in:

$$\dot{m}_t - \dot{m}_b \pm \dot{m}_p = C_m \frac{dP_m}{dt} \tag{3-20}$$

where mask capacitance $C_m = V_m/R_a T_m$.

The prediction of the bias airflow behavior through the vent holes is based on the pressure difference between the mask pressure (P_m) and atmospheric pressure (P_a). The relationship between the pressure difference and the flow rate through these vent holes can be written as [3]

$$P_m - P_a = \frac{\rho_a}{2C_d^2 A_b^2} Q_b^2 \tag{3-21}$$

where ρ_a is the density of the air contained within the mask; A_b is the minimum area of the bias vent hole; C_d *is* the discharge coefficient; and Q_b is the vent volume flow rate. The vent volume flow rate (Q_b) may be expressed as:

$$Q_b = \frac{\dot{m}_b}{\rho_a n} \tag{3-22}$$

where n is the number of holes venting air from the mask. Substituting equation (3-22) into equation (3-21) results in:

$$P_m - P_a = \frac{\dot{m}_b^2}{2C_d^2 A_b^2 - \rho_a n^2} \qquad (3-23)$$

Accurate determination of the nasal mask vent flow discharge coefficient (C_d) is difficult since the number of holes varies with mask design and manufacturer. These holes are physically characterized as being a combination of a sharp-edged orifice and a sudden expansion into open space. However, these holes are usually of tapering diameter and short length. In this chapter a loss coefficient C_d of 0.8 is assumed, which is between the coefficient for a sudden expansion ($C_d = 1$) and a sharp-edged hole ($C_d = 0.6$).

The mask vent relationship is nonlinear, so to linearize this behavior, a reference point of 10 cm H_2O is considered, which is between the normal operating pressure range of 6 to 20 cm H_2O [4], producing an error of –6 to +5%.

The mask vent bias flow can now be represented by:

$$P_m - P_a = R_b \dot{m}_b + Y_b \qquad (3-24)$$

where R_b is the gradient of the linearized flow characteristic; and Y_b represents the y intercept.

Rearranging equation (3-24) and substituting into equation (3-20) gives an expression that enables mask pressure to be expressed in terms of supply tube and patient breathing air mass flow rates:

$$\dot{m}_t - \left(\frac{P_m - P_a - Y_b}{R_b} \right) \pm \dot{m}_p = C_m D P_m \qquad (3-25)$$

where mask capacitance $C_m = V_m / R_a T_m$.

Rearranging equation (3-25) yields the following expression, which can be used to model the breathing system mask pressure:

$$\frac{P_m}{\dot{m}_t + \frac{P_a}{R_b} + \dot{m}_p \frac{Y_b}{R_b}} = \frac{R_b}{R_b C_m D + 1} \qquad (3-26)$$

3.3 SIMULINK™ MODEL

The four main CPAP system elements, consisting of the air delivery unit, reservoir, delivery tube, and nasal mask can now be integrated into a complete breathing system model. A computer simulation model of the proposed breathing system is developed, in Simulink™ within the Matlab™ environment, utilizing an idealized air delivery unit. The governing equations used within the model simulation are detailed through the use of block diagram algebra (Figure 3-11) [1].

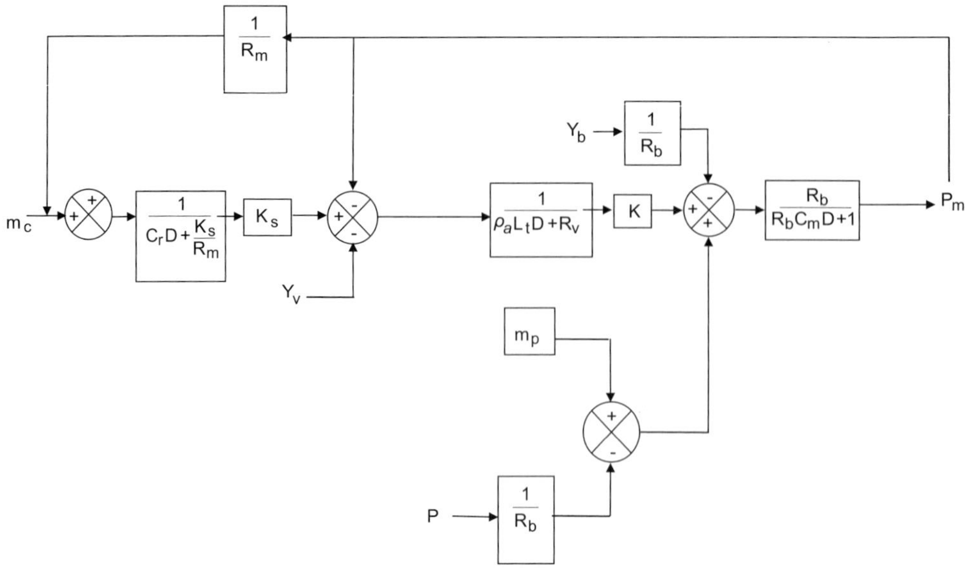

Figure 3-11. Block diagram of breathing system model [1]

The complete Simulink™ model (Figure 3-12) shows the breathing system divided into three main sections: the air delivery unit, reservoir and delivery tube, and the nasal mask. Closed loop pressure feedback control of the system is utilized to control the mask pressure fluctuations during patient breathing. Model pressure and mass flow rates are simulated to compare with a prototype breathing system.

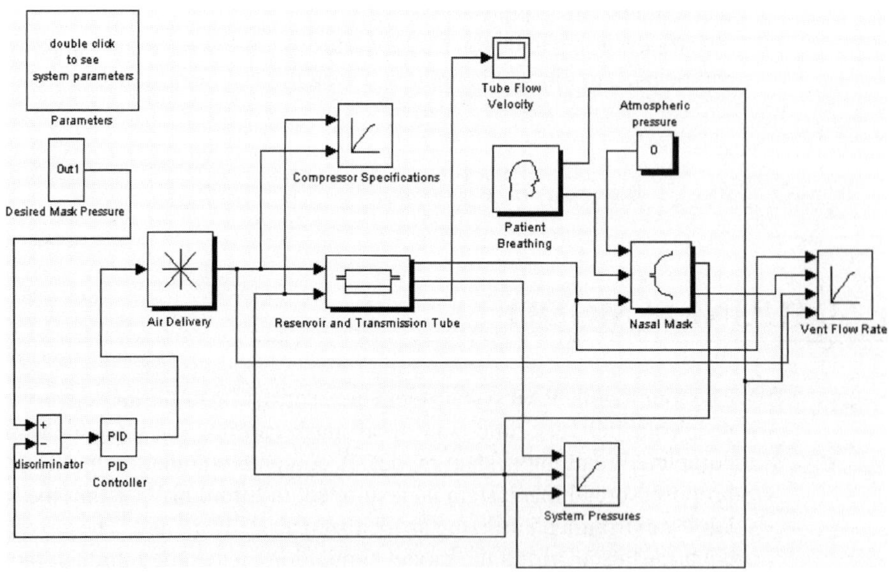

Figure 3-12. Simulink™ model of the CPAP breathing system

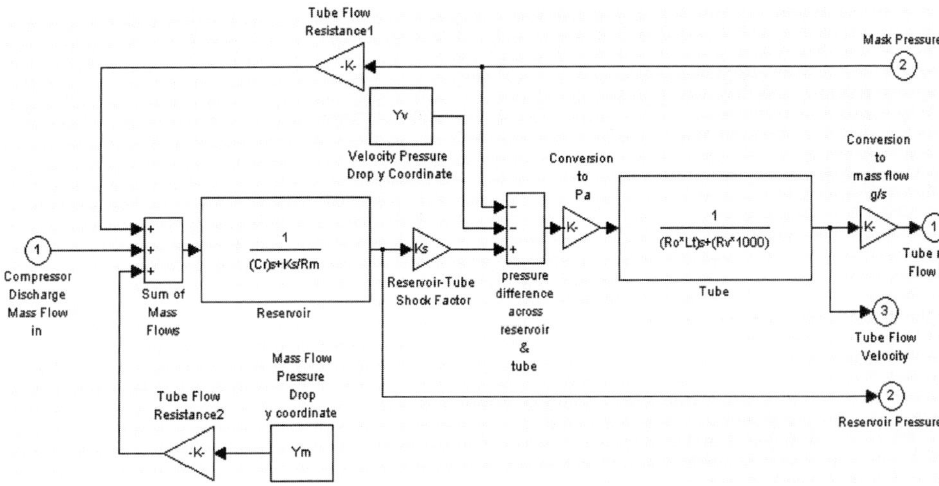

Figure 3-13. Simulink™ model of reservoir and delivery tube

The reservoir and delivery tube model elements (Figure 3-13) are combined into one model simulation block to simplify construction. Provision is made to input the prototype breathing system physical parameters into the combined reservoir-delivery tube model simulation element.

The mask model element simulation (Figure 3-14) consists of inputs from the delivery tube air inflow, patient breathing, and the mask vent outflow. Provision is also made here to input the physical parameters of the prototype breathing system into the mask model simulation element.

The patient breathing load (Figure 3-5) is inputted into the model simulation as an independent variable, read from a text file, representing the relaxed breathing cycle typical of a sleeping adult patient. Patient breathing air mass flow rate (g/s) is shown as a function of time; inhalation and exhalation being given as a positive and negative quantity, respectively.

3.4 MODEL VALIDATION

To validate a model that studies system dynamics, some standard procedures with standard inputs are normally used. These standard inputs include, but are not limited to, step, impulse, ramp, terminated ramp, and sinusoidal functions. Selection of any of these inputs must be experimentally accessible in order to achieve an appropriate validation. In this section a simple widely used step function input is used. This function is extremely useful for studying the effect of parameter changes in a given system or for comparing the relative performance of two different systems. Although a perfect step function is physically unrealizable, a system disturbance similar in nature is adequate to compare overall system response.

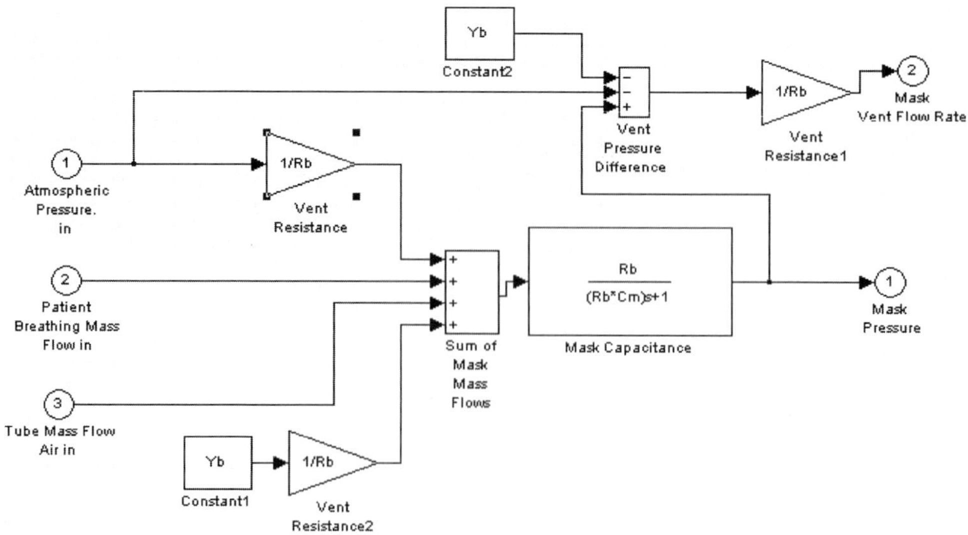

Figure 3-14. Simulink™ model of mask

White [1] developed and built an experimental setup to validate the step response for the reservoir and delivery tube model (Figure 3-13). The dynamic behavior of the prototype system is determined by introducing an airflow disturbance into the reservoir during operation of the system to produce a corresponding dynamic response in mask air pressure.

The flow signal for the breathing system is achieved by utilizing two air pressure regulators, connected in parallel, to supply air to the system reservoir (Figure 3-15) [1]. Each pressure regulator is preset to produce a steady state mask pressure within the system of 8 to 18 cm H_2O for the

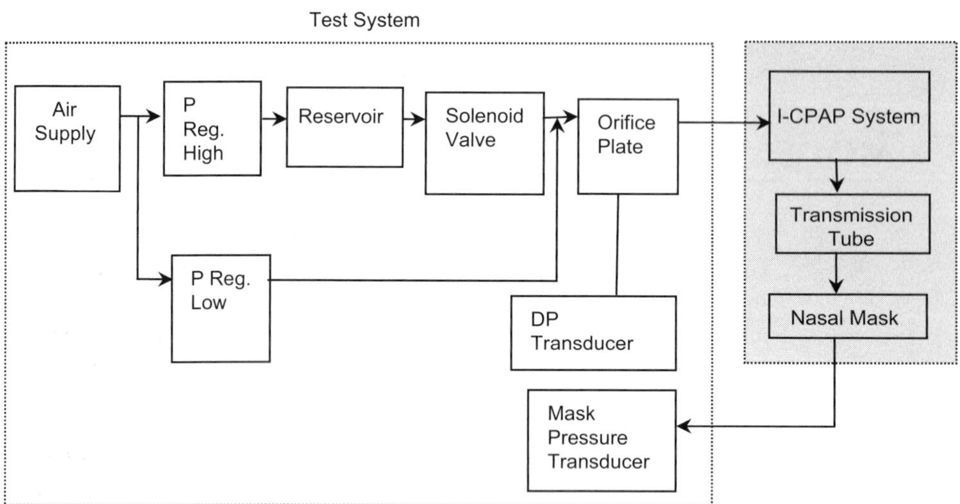

Figure 3-15. Schematic representation of prototype CPAP system test setup [1]

low and high pressure settings, respectively. Both low and high pressure regulator airflows pass through an orifice plate, which is used to measure the air mass flow into the prototype system reservoir. The low pressure regulator constantly supplies the nasal mask while the high pressure regulator is isolated from the system by a solenoid valve. Actuating the solenoid valve permits the higher pressure supply air to enter the system reservoir while the low pressure regulator, sensing the increase in downstream pressure, shuts off its air supply. The high pressure regulator is connected to a 6 L air reservoir, which provides additional high pressure air capacitance in order to minimize the fluctuation in supply air pressure when the solenoid valve is opened.

The signal input air mass flow rate measured by means of the orifice plate and differential pressure (DP) transducer is recorded for later use as an input air disturbance within the model. The system's mask air pressure response to the incoming air signal is measured and recorded by a pressure transducer. Both the measured signal disturbance and resultant mask air pressure fluctuation are delayed one second after model initiation, to ensure that the simulation is in equilibrium prior to the measured signal being input into the system. This ensures that any transient behavior in the model simulation, due to the initial starting and filling conditions, does not coincide with the time period where dynamic testing occurs.

Model simulation parameters are used from Table 3-1 [1] in the operation of the model, with the airflow disturbance being read from data obtained during testing of the prototype system. Figure 3-16 shows the experimental and the model prediction results. Both the steady state values and dynamic response behavior of the model compare very favorably with that of the actual breathing system tested. However, the measured system mask pressure response is slower than the model by about 20 ms,

TABLE 3-1. Computer simulation parameters

Element	Parameter	Value	Units
Reservoir	Capacitance	0.005604	g/kPa
	Shock Factor into Tube	0.9	
	Internal Diameter	5.5	mm
	Length	1.8	m
	Tube velocity pressure drop gradient	0.3752	kPa/ms^{-1}
Tube	Tube velocity pressure drop Y coordinate	–4.6587	kPa
	Tube mass flow pressure drop gradient	12.147	kPa/ms^{-1}
	Tube mass flow pressure drop Y coordinate	–4.6587	kPa
Air Properties	Average air density	1.334	kg/m^3
	Effective air bulk modulus	136330	Pa
	Capacitance	0.0011768	g/kPa
Nasal Mask	Bias mass airflow pressure drop gradient	3.3483	kPa/m/s
	Bias mass airflow Y coordinate	–0.981	kPa

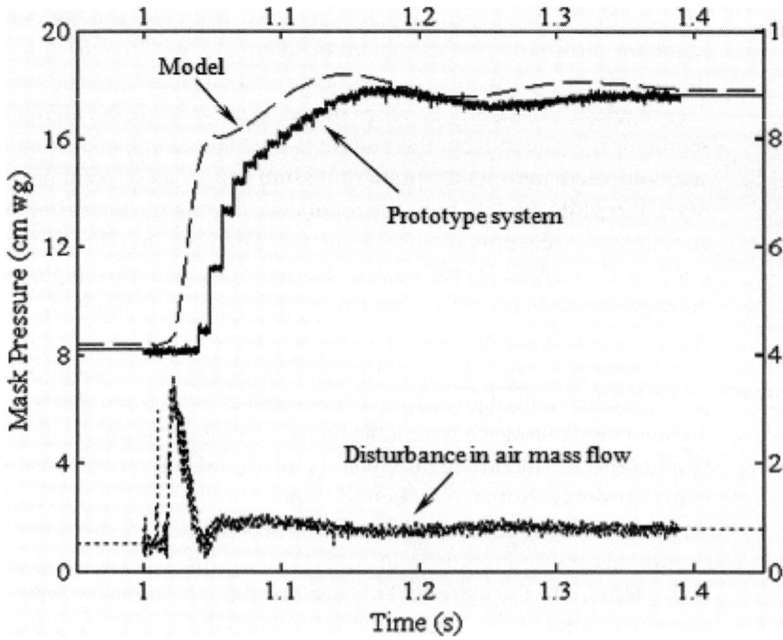

Figure 3-16. System and model simulation dynamic test response

which may be attributed to response delay times in measurement equipment that are not incorporated into the model. The signal interference spike in the input air mass flow at the 1.01-second interval is believed to be due to electromagnetic interference from the high pressure supply solenoid air valve and does not represent measured air mass flow.

The above validation indicates that the model does reasonably mimic the response of the actual system. This reflects a useful fact, showing that even with the many assumptions and simplifications to the real system, this modeling approach is very useful not only in showing the trend of behavior, but also in determining system performance under various system parameters as presented in the application in Section 3.5.

Once satisfied that the model is able to closely mimic the behavior of the actual system, it can be used to predict the air output specifications of a prototype system's elements, such as the compressor, or to assess the system performance when system parameters are changed for optimization or improvement purposes.

3.5 MODEL UTILITY

Assuming that use of the above model is required to assess the performance of a reciprocating compressor designed for this application, it is desirable to see how the proposed compressor affects the system performance when certain design parameters are changed. This is a very useful process in the preliminary stage of development and design.

It is extremely important to maintain the air pressure in the mask at the desired level within ± 0.5 cm H_2O or 0.05 kPa. The compressor that will be utilized in the system is a high speed, variable stroke reciprocating compressor with a single acting piston. It is believed that the compressor stroke can be changed from 0 to 12 mm on a per stroke basis, and reciprocates at around 200 cycles/s. The controller should thus be capable of controlling the piston stroke in each cycle, to maintain the desired pressure level in the mask with the specified limits.

3.5.1 Compressor Analysis

The compressor is a reciprocating type single acting machine with a variable stroke. As mentioned above, the stroke can be controlled for each cycle from 0 to 12 mm. Since the details of the mechanism by which the stroke is controlled are not available, it is assumed that the crank length is changed, while the length of the connecting rod of the piston is kept constant. Figure 3-17 illustrates the principle of a variable stroke reciprocating compressor. S_{max} and S are maximum stroke and any stroke, $V_{c,min}$ and V_c represent the corresponding clearance volumes, respectively. The compressor is modeled as an instantaneous element of the system. This means that the input-output characteristics of the compressor can be described by a set of algebraic equations. This assumption is justified as the compressor' dynamics are much faster (speed of rotation is around 200 cps) than the dynamics of the rest of the system.

Figure 3-18 depicts the thermodynamic cycle of a reciprocating compressor for a given stroke. P_d, P_s, and V_c, V_s are discharge and suction pressures and clearance and swept volumes of the compressor, respectively. It is assumed that for each cycle, the mass of air sucked at the suction pressure (P_s) is equal to the mass of air discharged at the discharged pressure (P_d). Thus, the mass discharged per cycle (m_d) is

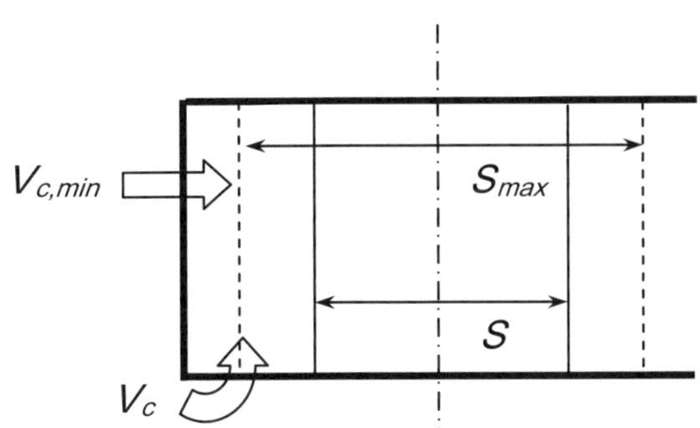

Figure 3-17. Principle of variable stroke reciprocating compressor

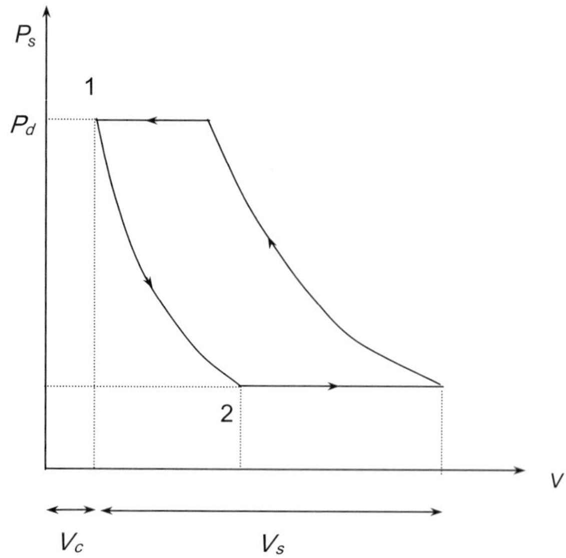

Figure 3-18. Thermodynamic cycle of a reciprocating compressor for a given stroke

given by:

$$m_d = \eta_v V_s \rho_a \qquad (3-27)$$

where V_s is the ideal volumetric efficiency; and ρ_a is the density of air, which is assumed to be independent of the pressure. The ideal volumetric efficiency (η_v) of a reciprocating compressor is defined as:

$$\eta_v = \frac{\text{The actual volume sucked}}{\text{The swept volume}} \qquad (3-28)$$

Based on the thermodynamic cycle in Figure 3-18, it can be shown that the ideal volumetric efficiency of the compressor can be mathematically expressed in terms of geometrical and thermophysical parameters of the system as follows:

$$\eta_v = 1 + C - C\left(\frac{P_d}{P_s}\right)^{\frac{1}{\gamma}} \qquad (3-29)$$

where C is the clearance fraction given by V_c/V_s; and γ is the ratio of the specific heats of air as expansion and compression processes are assumed to be isentropic. Since the clearance fraction is the ratio between the clearance and the swept volumes, which change with the stroke (See

Figure 3-17), the clearance fraction of a variable stroke compressor can be given by:

$$C = \frac{C_{min}S_{max} + 0.5S_{max}}{S} + (-0.5) = \frac{K_1}{S} + K_2 \qquad (3-30)$$

Note that for a given compressor S_{max} and C_{min} are constants and $C_{min} = \frac{V_{c,min}}{A_c S_{max}}$, where A_c is the cylinder bore area.

Since no information about the minimum clearance fraction is available, a value of 5% is assumed. Physical dimensions of the compressor are as follows:

- Cylinder bore (D_c) = 24 mm
- Maximum stroke (S_{max}) = 12 mm

Combining equations (3-27) to (3-29) leads to:

$$m_d = A_c\rho_a K_1 + (A_c\rho + A_c\rho K_2)S + \left(-\frac{K_1 A_c \rho}{P_s^{\frac{1}{\gamma}}} \right) P_d^{\frac{1}{\gamma}} + \left(-\frac{K_2 A_c \rho}{P_s^{\frac{1}{\gamma}}} \right) S\, P_d^{\frac{1}{\gamma}} \qquad (3-31)$$

In this equation the suction pressure (P_s) is equal to the atmospheric pressure, which is a constant. Thus, from a control point of view, the inputs to the compressor are the stroke (S) and the discharge pressure (P_d), and the output is the discharge mass flow per cycle (m_d). A more detailed discussion will be presented at a later stage when the analysis of the control system is considered.

3.5.2 System Model Summary

For clarity, component models developed above are tuned to the current application and summarized below.

$$m_d = A_c\rho_a K_1 + (A_c\rho_a + A_c\rho_a K_2)S + \left(-\frac{K_1 A_c \rho_a}{P_s^{\frac{1}{\gamma}}} \right) P_d^{\frac{1}{\gamma}} + \left(-\frac{K_2 A_c \rho_a}{P_s^{\frac{1}{\gamma}}} \right) S\, P_d^{\frac{1}{\gamma}} \qquad \text{Compressor}$$

$$\dot{m}_d = \frac{P_d - P_r}{R_d} \qquad \text{Discharge line}$$

$$\dot{m}_d - \dot{m}_s = \frac{dM_r}{d\theta} \qquad \text{Reservoir}$$

$$M_r = C_r P_r \qquad \text{Reservoir}$$

$$\dot{m}_s = \frac{P_r - P_m}{R_s} \qquad \text{Supply line}$$

$$\dot{m}_s - \dot{m}_v \pm \dot{m}_b = \frac{dM_m}{d\theta} \qquad \text{Mask}$$

$$M_m = C_m P_m \qquad \text{Mask}$$

$$\dot{m}_p = f(t) \qquad \text{Breathing}$$

$$\dot{m}_v = \frac{P_m - P_a}{R_v} \qquad \text{Ventilation}$$

For the controller, a proportional-integral and derivative (PID) controller is assumed

$$S = K_p e + T_i \int e.d\theta + T_d \frac{de}{d\theta} \qquad \text{Controller}$$

where S is the stroke of the compressor; and e is the error signal to the controller, which is equal to the difference between desired and measured values of the controlled variable.

TABLE 3-2. System constants

Constant	Description	Value	Units
A_c	Bore area	452.4	mm^2
S_{max}	Maximum stroke	12	mm
C_{min}	Minimum clearance ratio	5%	
P_a	Atmospheric pressure	101.3	kPa
$\bar{\dot{m}}_d$	Mean discharge/supply flow	08	gs^{-1}
R_d	Discharge line resistance	0.75	kPa/gs^{-1}
$\bar{P}_r$	Mean reservoir pressure	122.0	kPa
V_r	Reservoir volume	400.0	cm^3
C_r	Reservoir capacitance	0.00118	g/kPa
R_s	Supply line resistance	24.75	kPa/gs^{-1}
V_m	Mask volume	300.0	cm^3
C_m	Mask capacitance	0.00354	g/kPa
R_v	Ventilation hole resistance	1.125	kPa/gs^{-1}
P_m	Mean mask pressure	102.2	kPa
T	Air temperature	20.0	°C

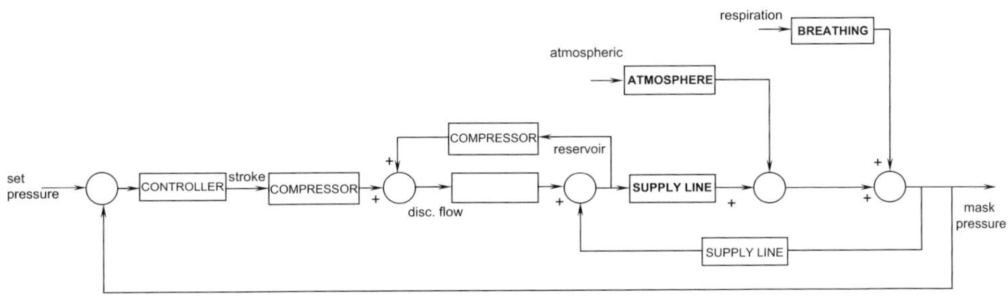

Figure 3-19. Block diagram of the system

Table 3-2 gives the system constants (including thermophysical parameters) that are used to simulate the overall model. A block diagram is developed in Figure 3-19 and a Simulink™ model is developed in Figure 3-20. It is to be noted that the mask pressure is the controlled variable, which has to be maintained within specified limits.

3.5.3 Simulation Results

In this section some important inferences from the model simulation results are presented. It is possible to look at the results for various parameters, but in this case, the compressor speed and mask and reservoir capacitances are chosen as the main parameters to investigate.

Figures 3-21 to 3-23 illustrate the dependence of the mask pressure, reservoir pressure, and compressor stroke on the compressor speed. Sim-

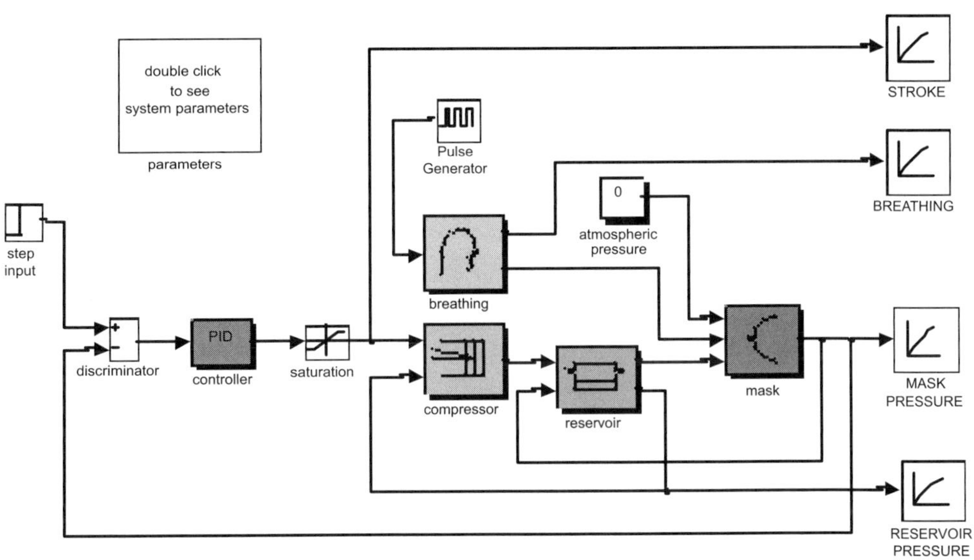

Figure 3-20. System simulink™ model

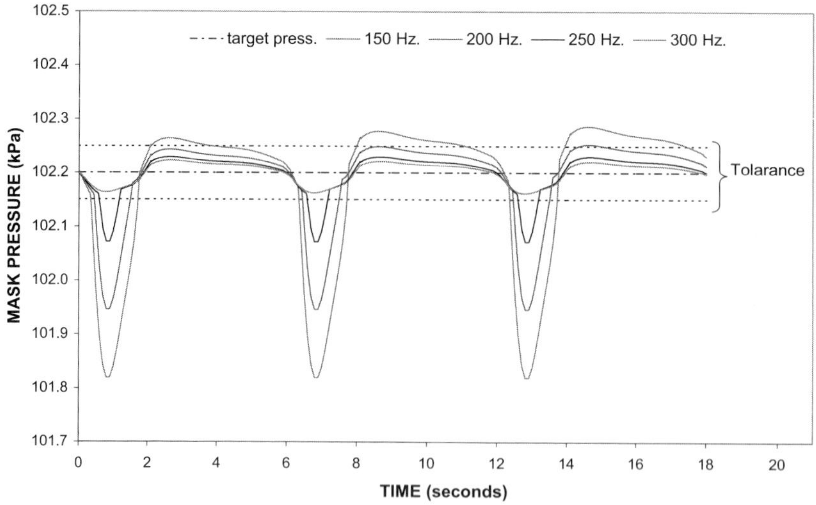

Figure 3-21. Mask pressure at different compressor speeds

ulations were carried out with controller parameters K_p = 100 mm/kPa; T_i = 10 s, and T_d = 0 s. It can be seen from Figure 3-21 that the compressor speed has to be maintained around 300 Hz in order to maintain the mask pressure within the specified limits. Compressor speed below this level causes the stroke to reach its upper saturation value of 12 mm (Figure 3-22). In the first half of the breath cycle (Figure 3-5), due to inhalation, there is a depletion of air resulting in a drop in the mask pressure.

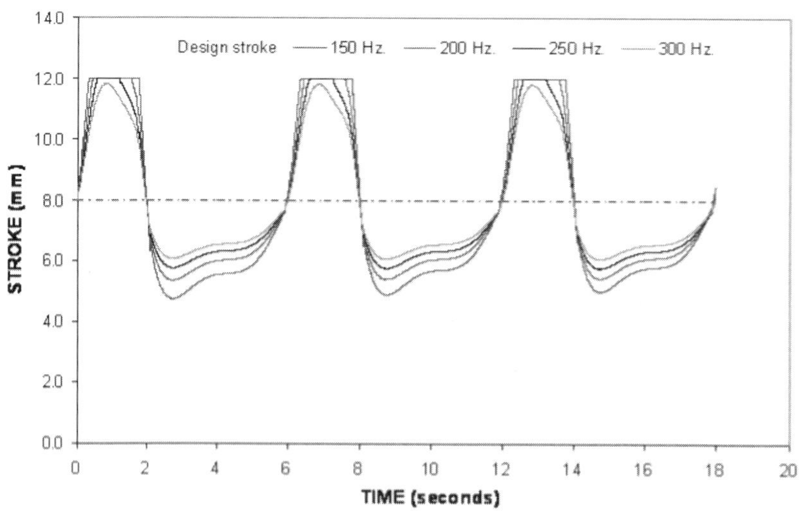

Figure 3-22. Compressor stroke at different compressor speeds

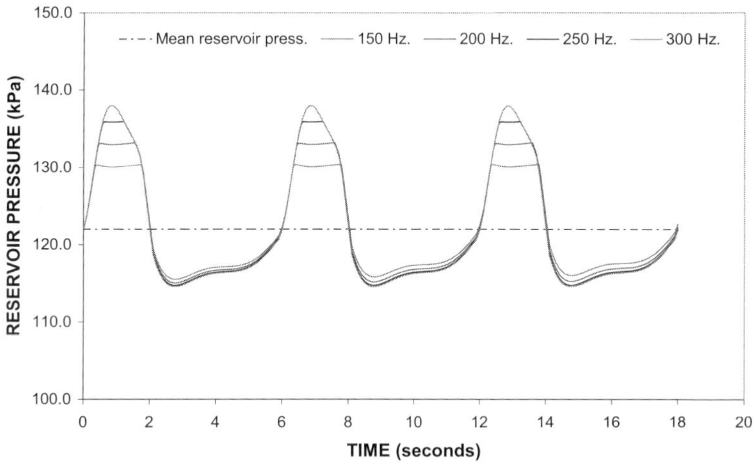

Figure 3-23. Reservoir pressure at different compressor speeds

The pressure drop is then transmitted to the controller and the stroke is increased accordingly. However, due to the upper saturation limit of the compressor stroke, the required amount of air cannot be supplied, and hence the pressure in the mask drops considerably below the targeted or desired pressure. The other interesting feature of the system is the amplitude of fluctuations in the reservoir pressure with compressor speed. Although the desired pressure level in the mask could be achieved with high rotational speeds, high rotational speeds cause the reservoir pressure to fluctuate with higher amplitudes (Figure 3-23). However, this phenomenon does not seem to have any negative impact on the mask pressure.

It is worthwhile to investigate the impact of the capacitances associated with the reservoir and mask on the system response. Figure 3-24 depicts how compressor stroke responds to the change in the reservoir capacitance. It is to be noted that the capacitance of the reservoir is a measure of its volume. The design value of the reservoir capacitance is 0.00118 g/kPa and the simulations were carried out at a compressor speed of 200 Hz, with the controller parameters set to 100.0 mm/kPa and 10 s for proportional gain and integral time, respectively. It can be seen from Figure 3-24 that the controller shows unstable behavior when the capacitance is about one-tenth of the design value. Figure 3-25 shows the same simulation with a magnified time scale. It is also noted from Figure 3-24 that as the capacitance of the reservoir increases, the response of the controller does not deteriorate. Figure 3-26 depicts a similar simulation with different values for the mask capacitance. In this simulation the mask pressure has been selected to illustrate the system response. It can be seen from Figure 3-26 that the mask capacitance does not affect the system response at all.

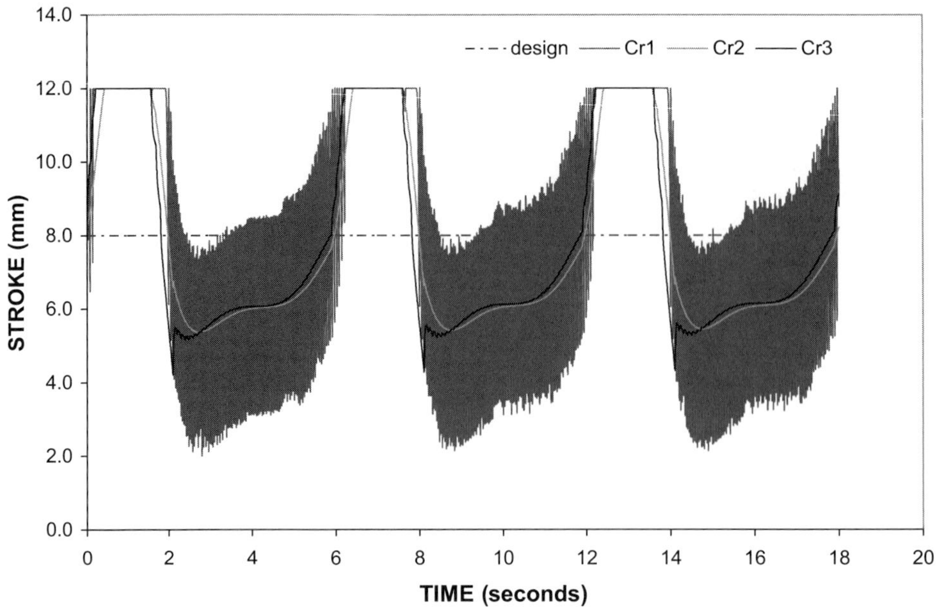

Figure 3-24. Effect of reservoir capacitance on stroke: C_{r1} = 0.0001 C_{r2} = 0.00118 and C_{r3} = 0.01 g/kPa

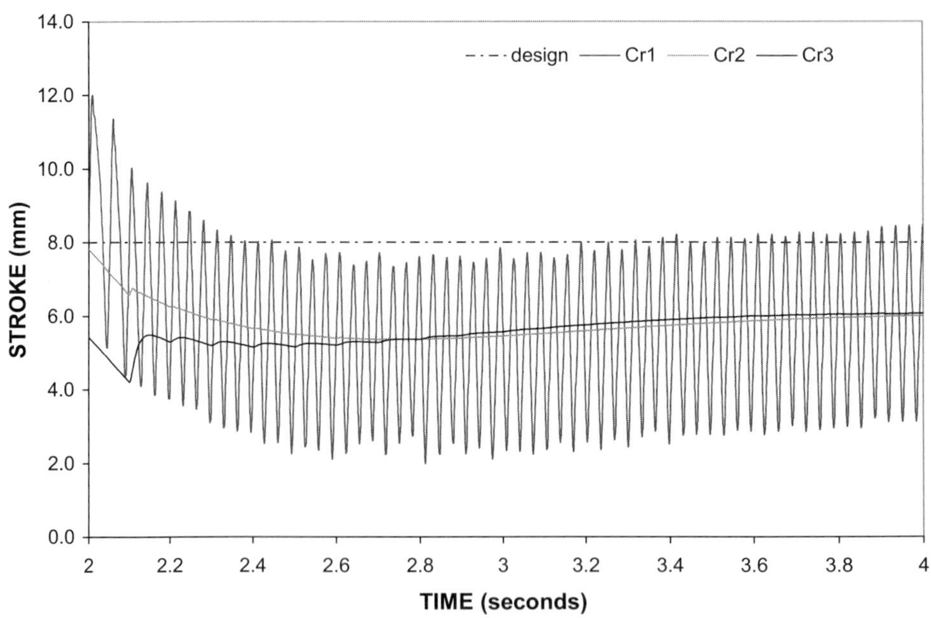

Figure 3-25. Stroke response at different mask capacitance (magnified time scale): Cr_1 = 0.0001 Cr_2 = 0.00118 and C_{r3} = 0.01 g/kPa

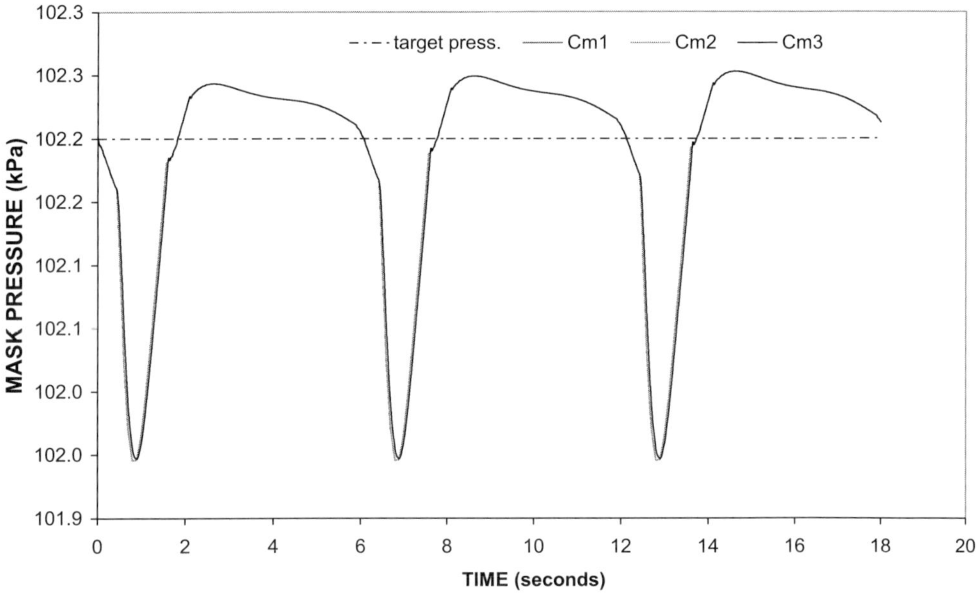

Figure 3-26. Effect of mask capacitance on system: C_{m1} = 0.001 C_{m2} = 0.00354 and C_{m3} = 0.0354 g/kPa

Subject to certain simplifying assumptions, a dynamic model was developed to simulate an artificial breather consisting of a single-acting-variable stroke reciprocating compressor, a reservoir, and a mask. The assumptions were:

1. Constant temperature of air.
2. Constant flow resistance through tubes.
3. No mass transfer (water evaporation) into the air stream.
4. No accumulation due to compressibility of air in the tubes.
5. Instantaneous input-output characteristics of the compressor.

The model governing equations were included in a Simulink™ model and are capable of simulating various system parameters, which are of interest from a control point of view. Some of the important conclusions drawn from the simulation are:

1. The compressor speed has to be at least 300 Hz if the maximum stroke is limited to 12 mm.
2. The reservoir capacitance (or size of the reservoir) does have a significant effect on the controller stability.
3. The mask capacitance does not show any significant effect on the system response.

3.6 REVERSED FLOW

Under some operating conditions, such as low CPAP pressure and/or high exhalation, some of the exhaled air will travel back into the delivery tube. Reverse flow occurs when the volumetric flow rate of the patient's exhalation is greater than the bias vent flow rate, so the pressure in the mask increases. The distance the exhaled air travels back into the Heated Air Delivery Tube (HADT) is defined as the distance of the reverse flow. This leads to fully saturated air at about 33°C that could produce condensation and raise the carbon dioxide concentration in the next inhalation. This section sets up a general mathematical model simulating this phenomenon. This will be helpful in the design and control development of a CPAP machine, and will eventually benefit users by reducing the possibility of condensation and carbon dioxide inhalation. The model should be able to quantify the reverse flow under a combination of pressure settings and breathing loads.

The distance for the reverse flow can be calculated by integrating the possible negative velocity V_t in each breath cycle:

$$\text{Distance travelled} = \int V_t dt \qquad (3-32)$$

where $V_t < 0$, and the integration range is repetitive within $n \cdot t_c < t < (n+1) \cdot t_c$ for each breath cycle, while $n = 0,1,2 \ldots$

The forward and reverse flow in the HADT is simplified by assuming that they displace each other. Although there might be some mixing of fresh air and exhaled air near the interface, it is not expected to significantly influence the condensation and CO_2 in the re-breath.

To determine an expression for the reversed flow velocity, an expression for the fluid velocity is developed. Knowing that $\dot{m}_t = \rho_a A_t V_t$, equation (3-7) can be rewritten as:

$$P_f = \frac{f - \rho_a L_t V_t^2}{2d_t} \qquad (3-33)$$

The forces exerted on the controlled volume include axial pressure generating forces on both ends and frictional force on the interface between the tube wall and the control volume. Thus, equation (3-6) above can be rewritten as:

$$\Delta P = -\rho_a A_t L_t \frac{dV_t}{dt} + P_f A_t \qquad (3-34)$$

where ΔP is the instantaneous fluctuating pressure drop over the tube length L_t as a result of the velocity fluctuation. For the model to be able to cope with positive and negative velocity, i.e., reverse flow, term V_t^2 in equation (3-33) may be rewritten as $V_t|V_t|$, so V_t alone can be used to determine the sign of this item and $V_t|V_t|$ together for value. Rearranging equation (3-34) gives:

$$\frac{dV_t}{dt} = \frac{\Delta P}{\rho_a L_t} - \frac{2f}{d_t} V_t|V_t| \qquad (3-35)$$

This equation is used to calculate the internal flow velocity fluctuation along with the change in pressure drop. If losses due to the outlet and inlet of the humidifier and the mask fittings, respectively, are considered, the total pressure drop can be written as their sum:

$$\Delta P_{losses} = \sum \frac{\rho_a k_i V_t^2}{2} \qquad (3-36)$$

where k_i is the minor heat loss coefficient, which is experimentally determined. Adding this to the right side of equation (3-34) gives the total pressure drop ΔP_{total} along the whole delivery tube from the reservoir to the mask, including friction and other losses:

$$\Delta P_{total} = \rho_a L_t \frac{dV_t}{dt} + \frac{2f}{d_t} V_t|V_t| + \sum \frac{\rho_a k_t V_t^2}{2} \qquad (3-37)$$

Therefore, to determine the velocity, the last equation can be written as:

$$\frac{dV_t}{dt} = \frac{\Delta P_{total}}{\rho_a L_t} - \left(\frac{2f}{d_t} + \frac{\sum k_i}{2L_t} \right) V_t|V_t| \qquad (3-38)$$

This equation can be used to calculate the internal flow velocity fluctuation in the tubing system with minor losses. However, if only the pressure drop due to friction with f as in equation (3-8) is considered and equation (3-8) is used, then the pressure at the mask P_M in terms of the pressure at the reservoir P_r can be written as:

$$P_M = \rho_a L_t \left[\frac{K_s P_r}{\rho_a L_t} - \frac{0.6328}{d_t \left(\frac{d_t -_a}{\mu} \right)^{0.25}} V_t|V_t| - \frac{dV_t}{dt} \right] \qquad (3-39)$$

where μ is the air viscosity. As shown above, the modeling process is identical to that in Section 3.2 with the exception of including the reverse flow in the equations. The rest of this section looks at the reversed flow in terms of its effect on transport delay, the air characteristics (fresh or re-breathed), and breathing load. Since modeling the whole process is too long to be included in this chapter, an example from the literature is summarized.

3.6.1 Transport Delay

In the delivery tube the air flow velocity fluctuates with time and can be negative when reverse flow occurs. That is to say, within a breath cycle, air is mainly flowing from the humidification reservoir toward the mask, then to the patient. However, for a short period of time within the cycle, it is possible that air is pushed back by exhalation from the mask toward the chamber. To analyze this, for a typical delivery tube of L_t m in length, the tube is divided into n lumps with each lump of length L_t/n cm. Due to the varying airflow velocity, the time of air flowing over one lump's length is also fluctuating. This fluctuating time may be from

$$dt = \frac{ds}{V_t} \qquad (3-40)$$

The in-tube airflow fluctuating velocity is a function of time. Inserting $s = \tilde{u}\,(t) \cdot t$ into equation (3-40) and integrating it yields:

$$t_t = \int_{L_t} \frac{dV_t.t}{V_t} \qquad (3-41)$$

where t_t is the varying transport delay for air flowing through a lump-long distance. For simplicity, a numerical approximation is used to calculate the varying transportation time:

$$t_t = \sum \Delta t = \frac{\Delta s}{V_t} \qquad (3-42)$$

3.6.2 Effect of Flow Direction on Air Properties

The transport of a fluid variable may be expressed by a simple expression as:
when $V_t > 0$

$$\lambda_n(t) = \lambda_{n-1}(t - t_1) \qquad (3-43)$$

and when $V_t < 0$

$$\lambda_n(t) = \lambda_{n+1}(t - t_1) \qquad (3-44)$$

where $\lambda_n(t)$ and $\lambda_{n-1}(t)$ are the airflow property fluctuation at lumps n and $n-1$, respectively. This indicates that if the variable has wavelength, it may experience a phase shift when transporting from one lump to another as indicated by equations (3-43) and (3-44).

As for airflow in the mask, the direction of transportation is controlled by the patient's respiration. Similar to the tube flow analysis during the inhalation phase, which is considered as positive flow, the transportation delay from the last lump of the HADT: (assuming 30 lumps in the tube model) to the mask is:

$$\lambda_M(t) = \lambda_{30}(t - t_1) \qquad (3-45)$$

Therefore, when there is a reverse flow, air comes from the mask into the last lump and the air properties of this lump will be:

$$\lambda_{30}(t) = \lambda_M(t - t_1) \qquad (3-46)$$

where $\lambda_{30}(t)$ and $\lambda_M(t)$ are the airflow's property fluctuation at lump 30 and the mask, respectively.

As for transportation between the reservoir and delivery tube lump 1: when $V_t > 0$

$$\lambda_1(t) = \lambda_C(t - t_1) \qquad (3-47)$$

and when $V_t < 0$

$$\lambda_C(t) = \lambda_1(t - t_1) \qquad (3-48)$$

where $\lambda_C(t)$ and $\lambda_1(t)$ are the airflow's property fluctuation in the reservoir and at lump 1, respectively.

3.6.3 Exhaled Air Re-breathing

If it is assumed that there is no bias flow through the mask vent holes with no reverse flow; the exhaled air should fill and stay in the mask and will be re-inhaled during the next inhalation process. However, when reverse flow occurs, in addition to the amount staying in the mask, part of the reversed exhaled air in the delivery tube may re-enter the mask at the start of the next inhalation and be re-inhaled. To determine the exhaled air re-breathing, it is necessary to consider the mixing of the fresh air and the exhaled air in the mask.

Two idealized models may be developed for the mixing process, one based on volume displacement and the other on perfect mixing. For the first one, when volume displacement occurs in the mask, a new volume of air enters the mask and pushes the previous fluid out of it. The gradual decrease in the amount of the previous volume in the mask can be expressed as:

$$C_t V_M = C_O V_M - \int \dot{q}_p dt \qquad 0 < C_O < 1, 0 < C_t < 1 \qquad (3-49)$$

where C_O is the volume concentration of the previous air in the mask at the beginning of the mixing; C_t is its gradually diluted volume concentration; $\dot{q}_p$ is the patient's respiratory volumetric flow rate; and V_M is volume capacity of the mask. Thus concentration (or ratio) of the previous fluid in the mask can be expressed as:

$$C_t = C_O\left(1 - \frac{\int \dot{q}_p dt}{V_M}\right) \qquad 0 < C_O < 1, 0 < C_t < 1 \qquad (3-50)$$

However, for perfect mixing, the new volume of air enters the mask and gets fully mixed with the previous volume and the mixture flows out with a continuously changing ratio of these two volumes. The concentration of the previous air in the mask will decrease following the formula below [5]:

$$C_t = C_O e^{\left(-\frac{\int \dot{q}_p dt}{V_M}\right)} \qquad 0 < C_O < 1, 0 < C_t < 1 \qquad (3-51)$$

In reality, mixing turns out to be somewhere between these two extremities: volume displacement and perfect mixing. That is to say that the concentration of the two types of air may decrease following a combination of the two expressions above, equations (3-50) and (3-51). If a ratio of 1:1 is chosen for the ratio of displacement to perfect mixing for the mixing in the mask, the combination of the two gives:

$$C_t = C_O\left[0.5\left(1 - \frac{\int \dot{q}_p dt}{V_M}\right) + 0.5 e^{\left(-\frac{\int \dot{q}_p dt}{V_M}\right)}\right] \qquad (3-52)$$

Equation (3-52) is drawn in Figure 3-27. This figure indicates that if mixing is expressed by this equation, then when the reversed air flows into the mask, the original exhaled air within the mask will be totally replaced after the reversed amount reaches about 1.3 times the mask capacity.

Mixing of exhaled air with fresh air in the mask may occur twice in a respiratory cycle, one starts at the beginning of inhalation and the other starts at the beginning of exhalation. When the exhalation phase begins, the concentration of fresh air already-in-mask decreases in accordance with the following expression [5]:

$$C_{MFet} = C_{MFeO}\left[0.5\left(1 - \frac{\int \dot{q}_p dt}{V_M}\right) + 0.5 e^{\left(-\frac{\int \dot{q}_p dt}{V_M}\right)}\right] \qquad (3-53)$$

While the concentration of exhaled air in the mask increases according to the formula:

$$C_{MEet} = 1 - C_{MFeO}\left[0.5\left(1 - \frac{\int \dot{q}_p dt}{V_M}\right) + 0.5 e^{\left(-\frac{\int \dot{q}_p dt}{V_M}\right)}\right] \qquad (3-54)$$

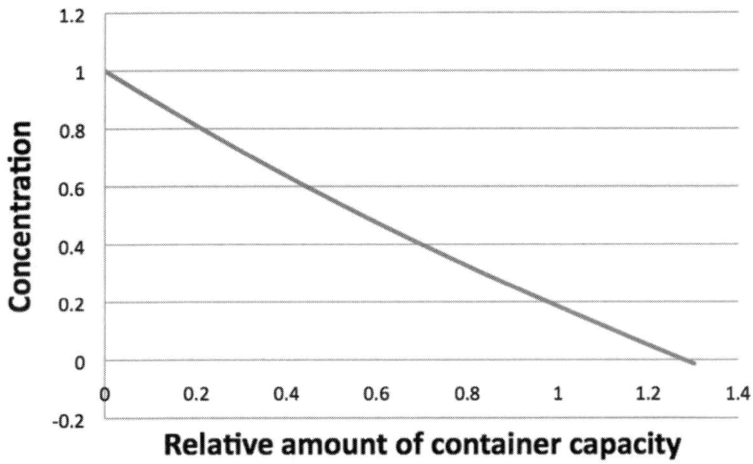

Figure 3-27. Reversed and exhaled air mixing curve in the mask

Alternatively, at the beginning of the inhalation phase, if the air coming from the delivery tube is fully fresh, the concentration of exhaled air decreases according to:

$$C_{MEit} = C_{MEiO}\left[0.5\left(1-\frac{\int \dot{q}_p dt}{V_M}\right)+0.5e^{\left(-\frac{\int \dot{q}_p dt}{V_M}\right)}\right] \qquad (3-55)$$

The percentage of exhaled air re-breathed within a total inhalation can be calculated by:

$$C_{Erb} = 100\% \times \frac{\int C_{ME}.\dot{q}_p dt}{\int \dot{q}_p dt} \qquad (3-56)$$

with integration only over the inhalation phase.

3.6.4 Modeling Outcomes

To determine the above parameters and the effect of the reversed flow, a typical tube length of 175 cm is considered. The tube is divided into 30 lumps with each lump of 5.75 cm, and Δs is taken as 1/10 of a lump length, i.e., 5.75 mm, which is small enough and may give a good approximation for this varying time span.

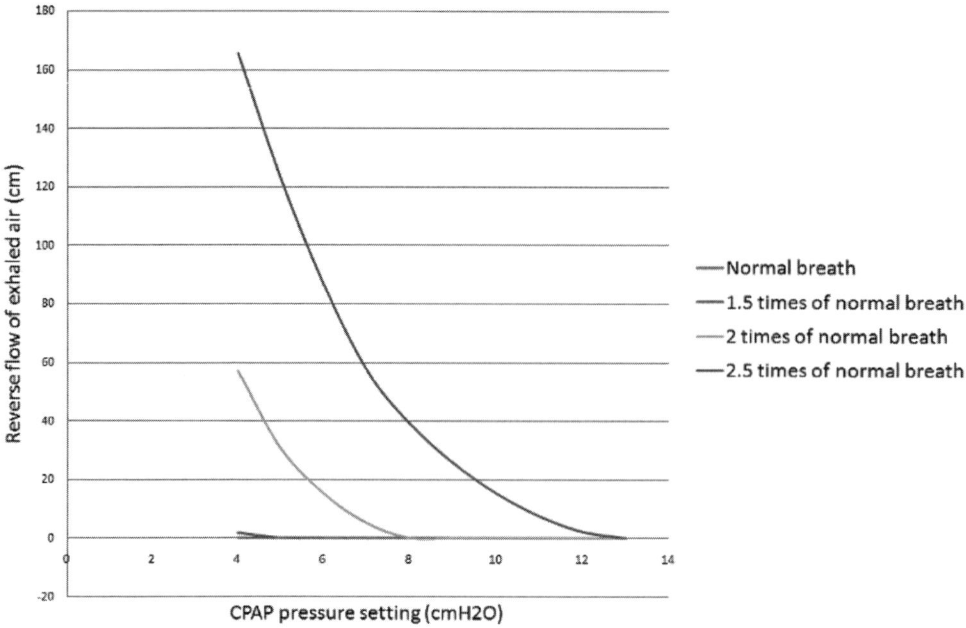

Figure 3-28. Reverse flow under different combinations of breath load and CPAP pressure setting [6]

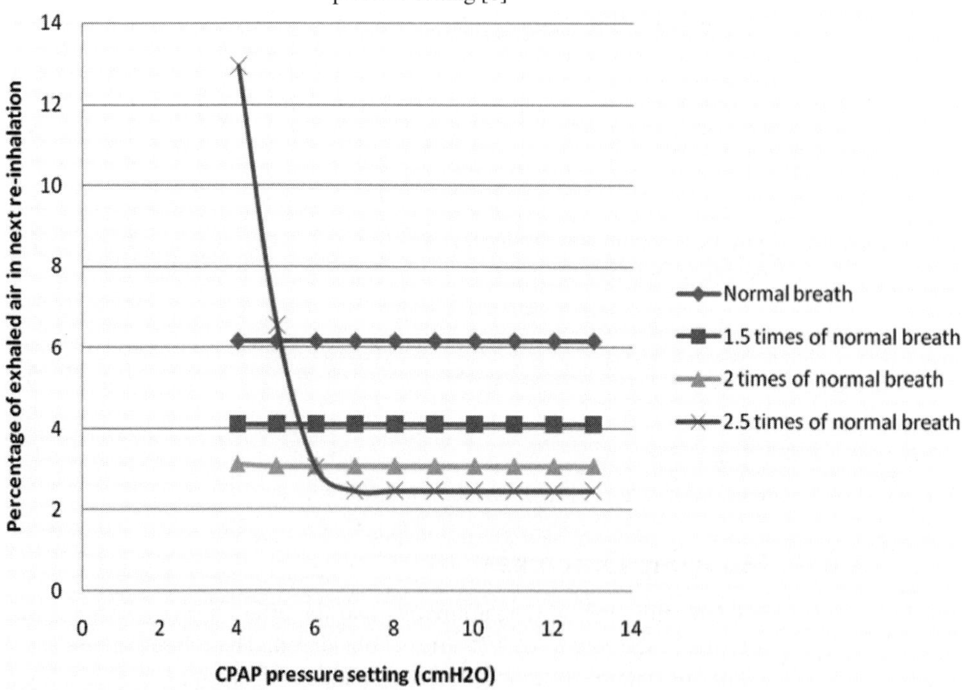

Figure 3-29. Percentage of exhaled air in inhalation under different combinations of breath load and CPAP pressure setting when using nasal mask

If the air from the delivery tube is not fully fresh (because of reverse flow), Equation (3-55) can give the concentration of decreasing exhaled air as:

$$C_{MEit} = C_{MEtO}\left[0.5\left(1-\frac{\int \dot{q}_p(1-C_{El30})dt}{V_M}\right)+0.5e^{\left(-\frac{\int \dot{q}_p(1-C_{El30})dt}{V_M}\right)}\right] \quad (3-57)$$

where C_{El30} is the exhaled air concentration in flow from lump 30 of the tube.

To determine the reverse flow, transport delay, and percentage of re-breathed exhaled air, equations (3-39) to (3-57) are implemented in the model developed in Li [6]. The results are summarized as follows:

1. In general, under normal breathing, there is no reverse flow. However, when the breath load is increased by 1.5, 2, and 2.5 times normal breathing under different CPAP pressure settings, the reverse flow outputs from the model are shown in Figure 3-28. This indicates that there is almost no reverse flow at 1.5 times normal breathing. Reverse flow is cut off at 8 cm H_2O and 13 cm H_2O for 2 and 2.5 times, respectively. Overall, when breath load increases, reverse flow increases and when the pressure setting increases, the reverse flow drops. The figure also shows that the distance of reverse flow is the same when mask capacity changes. This is attributed to the assumption of air incompressibility, which means that the distance of reverse flow is not influenced by the mask capacity.
2. Figure 3-29 shows the percentage of exhaled air inhalation versus comhbination of breath load and pressure settings at a nasal mask. Comparing this figure with Figure 3-28 indicates that reverse flow does not definitely increase exhaled air re-inhalation. When the breath load is 2 times normal breathing, reverse flow can occur until a pressure setting of 7 cm H_2O; however, re-inhalation only increases slightly when the pressure setting is at the lowest, 4 cm H_2O. When the breath load is 2.5 times normal breathing, reverse flow can occur when pressure is as high as 12 cm H_2O, but the re-inhalation increase vanishes when

TABLE 3-3. Ratio of percentage of exhaled air in inhalation between full-face mask and nasal mask [6]

Breath Load (Times of Normal Breathing)	Exhaled Air Re-breath (% in Inhalation)		Ratio of Full-Face/ Nasal Masks
	Nasal	Full-Face	
Normal	5.17	17.44	3.375
1.5	3.45	11.63	
2	2.58	8.72	
2.5	2.07	6.98	

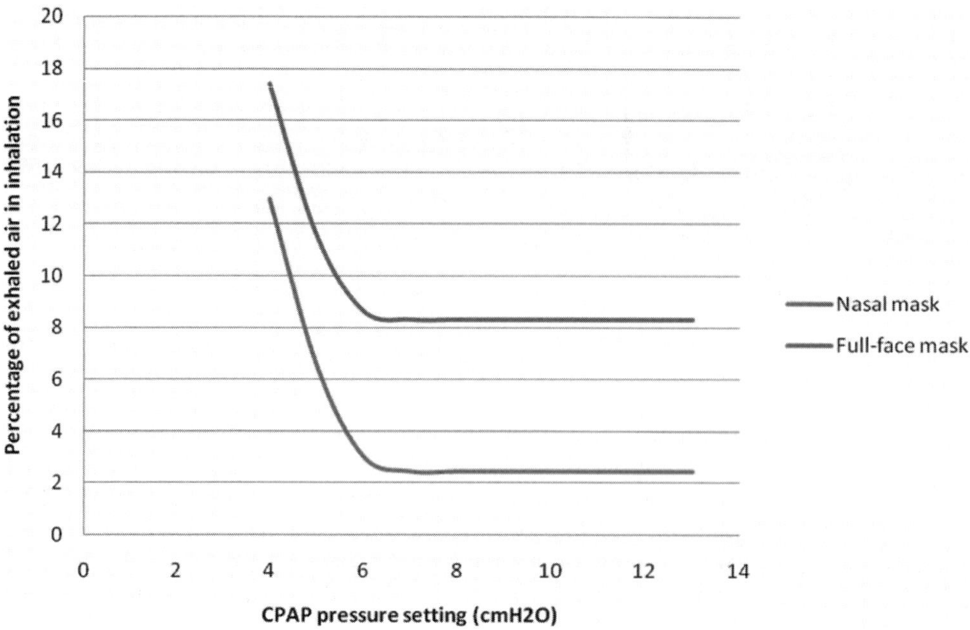

Figure 3-30. Comparison of exhaled air re-inhalation between nasal mask and full-face mask when there is reverse flow influence

pressure setting is above 6 cm H_2O. This is attributed to the fact that at the end of exhalation, the exhaling flow rate tends to be smaller than the bias vent flow rate, and the air from CPAP resumes moving toward the mask before the inhalation phase starts. Since inhalation has not started yet, the airflow can only flow out from the bias vent holes. If the exhaled air in the tube has already been completely expelled before the patient starts the next inhalation, the airflow entering the mask will be fully fresh. However, if the reverse flow is too far back into the tube when the breath load is large and the pressure setting is low, a certain amount of the in-the-tube exhaled air can re-enter the mask and can add to the re-inhalation. Figure 3-29 indicates that when the pressure setting is at 4 cm H_2O and the breath load is 2.5 times normal breathing, which is 2023 ml for one inhalation, the exhaled air remaining in the mask consists of 2.07% of the next inhalation. When exhaled air from reverse flow is added, it becomes 12.54% of the total volume of an inhalation. However, since the breath load rarely reaches 2000 ml, the reverse flow's influence on exhaled air re-inhalation is negligible.

3. When there is no exhaled air added in the mask from reverse flow, the re-inhaled air is only what is remaining in the mask. In this case the percentage of exhaled air in the next inhalation is proportional to mask capacity, as shown in Table 3-3. From this table, if the mask

capacity of a typical full-face mask is 236 ml and the breath load is normal, the percentage of exhaled air in the next inhalation process can reach above 17% and the volumetric percentage of CO_2 can reach about 0.87%, which is higher than the eight-hour time limit but lower than the 15-minute average limit of CPAP use. When the reverse flow adds exhaled air to the inhalation, the full-face mask also gives a higher percentage of exhaled air to the inhalation (Figure 3-30). This demonstrates that the mask capacity is a significant factor in influencing exhaled air re-breathing.

3.7 CLOSURE

This chapter presented the principle of operation of a CPAP system followed by modeling of its various components based on a systems modeling approach. The overall system model is then constructed and validated experimentally. A practical exercise is presented in Section 3.5 to show the effectiveness and utility of the simulation process. The process of reverse flow and its implications on CO_2 re-breathing and condensation are also discussed and modeled at the end of the chapter.

REFERENCES

[1] White, D.E., Breathing Therapy Air Delivery Unit: Simulation, Design and Development, Master of Engineering thesis, 2003. Auckland University of Technology, Auckland.

[2] Fox, R. and MacDonald, A., *Introduction to Fluid Mechanics*, 4th ed., 1994. John Wiley & Sons, New York.

[3] Streeter, V.L., Wylie, E.B., and Bedford, K.W., *Fluid Mechanics*, 9th ed., 1998. Mc-Graw-Hill, Singapore.

[4] Verse, T., Pirsig, W., Stuck, B., Hormann, K., and Maurer, J.T., Recent Developments in the Treatment of Obstructive Sleep Apnea. *Am J of RespMed*, 2003. **2**(2): p. 157–68.

[5] Newman, E.V., Merrell, M., Genecin, A., Monge, C., Milnor, W.R., and McKeever, W.P., The Dye Dilution Method for Describing the Central Circulation: An Analysis of Factors Shaping the Time-Concentration Curves. *Circulation*, 1951. **4**(5): p. 735–46.

[6] Li, C., The Effect of CPAP Tube Reverse Flow, Master of Engineering thesis, 2008. Auckland University of Technology, Auckland.

Chapter 4

MODELING CPAP HUMIDIFICATION

Modeling of the humidification process in a typical Continuous Positive Airway Pressure (CPAP) device is described in this chapter, by developing a model that predicts the mask absolute humidity level and air temperature due to the physical, mechanical, and thermodynamic behavior of individual elements. Such a model is formulated by incorporating the relationship between the inputs and measurable outputs in terms of air conditions at the mask. The system model inputs include machine settings and sensor readings.

Modeling a system in this fashion is shown to accurately predict the behavior of a typical system humidifier, heated air delivery tube, flexible tube, and nasal mask system elements.

4.1 THE NEED FOR HUMIDIFICATION

Normally air is inspired across a wide range of humidity levels and temperatures. Under CPAP treatment without humidification, the inspired air relative humidity level is normally around 24.0 ± 9.1 % and expired air is around 75.5 ± 14.4 % [1]. Before the inspired air reaches the isothermal saturation boundary (ISB), the point at which gases reach alveolar conditions (37°C and 100% relative humidity), the airway acts as a countercurrent heat and moisture exchanging system assisted by turbulent gas flow [2]. The inspired air gains heat and moisture from the upper airway lining, which is partly (one-third) restored when expired gas loses heat, and moisture condenses back to the airway surface [3, 4]. Normal condensation occurs in this case, because during expiration, the upper airway temperature always remains below the core body temperature. Breathing is related with a net heat and moisture loss because the expired air temperature and relative humidity are higher than the ambient conditions under most circumstances. In general, the greater the difference between the inspired and expired gas conditions, the higher the losses [4].

Clinical data suggests that the supply of gases at body temperature and pressure, saturated with water vapor (BTPS) of 37°C, containing 44 mg/L of water at approximately atmospheric pressure are optimal for the intubated patient [5, 6]. The International Organization of Standardization (ISO) recommends that inspiratory gas should possess a minimum absolute humidity of 33 mg/L [7]. ISO and the American National Standards Institute (ANSI) recommend that the absolute humidity level should be lower than 30 mg/L, as it is the minimum amount of water necessary to prevent the thickening of secretions and mucosal damage. With endotracheal intubation, the supply gas must be in "BTPS condition" because it bypasses most of the normal heat and moisture exchanging areas of the respiratory system [2].

For CPAP treatment, the inspired air relative humidity and temperature levels are dependent on the patient, as additional humidification can be expected from breathing through the nose [8]. The nasal mucosa has significant capacity to humidify the inspired air to reach BTPS conditions but this capacity can be overwhelmed at high flow rates, particularly under unidirectional flow (mouth leak) [3]. When the inspired gas humidity is low, evaporation occurs in the mucus, which makes it increasingly viscous. In this case, the cilia are unable to move the mucus, which cools down the trachea due to evaporation. The position of the ISB falls from typically the fourth or fifth generation of the subsegmental bronchi to the lower respiratory tract, which is poorly suited to heat and moisture exchange, resulting in cell damage and consequent infection [6].

A common side effect for patients using a CPAP device is a sore and dry nose and throat due to mouth leak, which occurs when the CPAP user sleeps with his/her mouth open. Instead of all of the air flowing down into the respiratory tract, some of it escapes through the oral cavity, which results in a decrease in the inspired air relative humidity level [3, 9, 10].

Mouth leak occurs in most users who suffer from dryness of nose and throat for approximately 31% of their total sleep time. Some of the pressurized air from the CPAP machine travels to the user's lung but a large portion of it leaks straight out from the mouth, which is called unidirectional flow. Studies on mouth leak showed that it increases the amount of nasal airway resistance (NAR), which results in nasal irritation and induced mouth breathing, creating a pathological circle [3].

4.2 TYPES OF HUMIDIFIERS

The three major types of humidification devices for CPAP therapy are heated humidifiers, passive humidifiers, and hygroscopic condenser humidifiers, which are explained in this section.

In the first type, the humidifier is connected within the CPAP system and has a heater plate temperature control. After the temperature is set, the heater plate heats up the water, to produce water vapor to humidify the pressurized air, and thus the air is humidified before it reaches the nose [11]. In comparison with heated humidifiers and passive humidifiers, the third type gives only a modest increase in the absolute humidity in the CPAP tube system and shows that considerably better results can be obtained with a heated humidifier [12]. The following sections give more details about these humidifiers.

4.2.1 Heated Humidifiers

In the heated humidification process, heating of water directly affects the humidity output of the humidification chamber [13]. Other factors that could affect the humidity of the inspired gas include the humidification chamber design and condensation along the inspiratory tubing [13]. The vaporizing capacity of a heated humidification chamber depends on the available water surface area [4, 14].

Observed variations in the heated humidifier performance in various environments suggest that specific external factors can affect the humidifier performance [5]. This is attributed to the fact that heated humidifiers do not have humidity control. Rather, they control the temperature and achieve humidification as a secondary effect. The humidity output from the humidifier chamber varies considerably when the inlet air temperature changes. It increases when the inlet gas temperature drops, which is attributed to the fact that when the cold air has been fed into the chamber, the control system has to increase the water temperature to maintain a constant chamber temperature. As described by Maxwell's speed distribution equation, the higher the temperature of the liquid, the higher the evaporation rate. This indicates that the evaporation rate of a heated humidifier is mainly dependent on water temperature. The observed effects of the ambient temperature on humidity output are related to the effect of the latter on the humidifier gas inlet temperature.

Heated humidifiers have a potential problem of output humidity level dropping when the inlet gas temperature rises. There are many factors that can affect the humidifier inlet air temperature such as the ambient temperature, the effect of ventilators, circuit length, and circuit insulation. It has been demonstrated that the heated humidifier performance drops with lower inlet air temperatures. An inlet temperature range from 16.6°C up to 40°C causes significant reduction in humidity [15]. This is attributed to the high inlet gas temperature raising the overall chamber temperature, which causes the control system to lower the water temperature to maintain the desired overall chamber temperature. It is also shown that flow and patient temperature variation does not affect the absolute humidity calculation [15].

Different environmental conditions affect the visible signs of humidity production, such as water loss in the chamber and the amount of condensation in the system. In some home care circumstances, this effect is exaggerated because the room temperature variation is larger than in a hospital.

Experimental investigations conducted on a CPAP humidifier have shown that the power consumption of the heater is proportional to the airflow rate through the humidifier, since a higher gas flow rate means a higher heat loss from the humidifier reservoir [16]. Theoretically, the humidifying efficiency depends on the amount of time that air is in contact with the reservoir surface. The greater the air volume flow rate, or minute ventilation, the smaller the resident time in the reservoir and the lower the humidifier performance [14]. The reservoir level inside the humidifier chamber has very little effect on power consumption. Also, the chamber reservoir level has no significant effect on the humidity production. Different humidifier reservoir chamber designs produce various ranges of humidity outputs for heated humidifiers [16].

As air flows out of the humidifier toward the patient in an unheated tube, it cools down, resulting in a large volume of condensation inside the tube [17]. This reduces the airflow absolute humidity (AH) level and may result in infection caused by inspiration of contaminated condensation [2, 4]. Another concern with water condensation in the air delivery tube is that it may become contaminated or interfere with the function of the ventilator [18]. Therefore, a heated-wire system in the air delivery tube was developed to eliminate the condensation and maintain a constant absolute humidity level [2]. The setting of the heated air delivery tube can alter the airflow temperature (and thus the airflow relative humidity) at the outlet of the tube. For a heated humidifier without a heated air delivery tube, the humidifier chamber temperature must be kept at 50°C in order to achieve 37°C air temperature at the patient end of the delivery tube [19]. However, if the airflow is heated higher than the humidification chamber temperature, it can reduce the relative humidity (RH) level, which may result in thickened secretions in the upper airway, especially in tracheostomy or endotracheal tubes [2]. It is worth mentioning that airflow in a saturation condition (100% RH) has no ability to absorb any water from the airway until it is warmed. Therefore, gases with high RH and low temperature will deprive the peripheral airway of water once the gases have been warmed due to the low AH level [2]. However, it was found that, with a reasonable range of temperature difference, which means less than 3°C higher than the saturation temperature, the reduction in relative humidity appears to be clinically unimportant. For air temperatures 3°C or more above the saturation temperature, the reduction of relative humidity can be low enough to cause drying of the airway and airway obstruction [19].

This type of a humidifier is the most commonly used and will be analyzed in detail in the following sections.

4.2.2 Passive Humidifiers

For passive humidification, the air passes through a container that is half-filled with water. Most passive humidifiers direct the pressurized air over a large surface area of water to increase the ability of the air to absorb as much moisture as possible. Both molecular water vapor and water droplets are added to the supply airflow from the ventilator. As the water is at room temperature, the pressurized air can only absorb small amounts of moisture as it passes over. Passive humidifiers have had growing acceptance in recent years due to their low cost, simple operation, and elimination of condensation in the circuit [20]. Therefore, humidifiers are suitable for patients who suffer from mild to moderate nasal congestion, or complain of difficulty breathing through the heated humidifier. Research has shown that passive humidifiers with high dead space may adversely affect respiratory function in certain patients [20]. A passive humidifier with increased dead space is associated with an increased dead space to tidal volume ratio [21], which can be expressed as:

$$\frac{V_D}{V_T} = \frac{P_{aCO_2} - P_{\bar{E}CO_2}}{P_{aCO_2}} \qquad (4-1)$$

where $P_{\bar{E}CO_2}$ is the mixed expired carbon dioxide; and P_{aCO_2} is the arterial partial pressure of carbon dioxide.

A passive humidifier with a large dead space may negatively impact the respiratory function of a spontaneously breathing patient, increasing respiratory rate and minute volume to maintain constant alveolar ventilation and arterial partial pressure of carbon dioxide. For a paralyzed patient, the larger ratio of dead space volume to tidal volume causes a small but statistically significant increase in arterial partial pressure of carbon dioxide [21]. To select a suitable passive humidifier, a clinician should be aware of the effect of the humidifier dead space on the patient's respiratory function.

In comparison, the heated and passive humidification modes both show significant increase in the inspired air RH level [1]. However, heated humidification is the only one that shows a clinically relevant increase in RH level [1]. Investigations have shown that the heated humidification mode had the lowest moisture loss [22]. As nasal obstruction is one of the major side effects of CPAP treatment, it is important to determine the influence of various modes of humidification in the impedance of upper airways.

4.2.3 Hygroscopic Condenser Humidifiers

Another type of humidification is the hygroscopic condenser humidifier (HCH), which uses small amounts of disposable hygroscopic materials (such as $CaCl_2$, $MgCl_2$, and LiCl) that trap heat and moisture from expired air and return it with the next inspiratory breath [4]. In this system, the expiration gas absolute humidity is related to the inspiration absolute humidity [1, 23]. An HCH insert fits between the patient's nose and the expiratory valve [8]. Experiments showed that by using HCHs in CPAP treatment, the relative humidity of inspired gas increased from 36.6 ± 4 to 63.1 ± 1.2% under an air pressure of 7.5 cm H_2O [8]. Portability is the main advantage of the HCH, but it is recommended that the humidifier be changed every 24 hours in mechanical ventilation to avoid bacterial contamination [8].

The active heat and moisture exchanger (AHME), shown in Figure 4-1, combines the passive operation of an HCH with additional heat and moisture supplied by a heater and water source [19]. An AHME component includes an HCH, a temperature and water control unit, a water unit, and a temperature probe. In this system, the HCH is modified by connecting it to the hygroscopically treated corrugated paper medium, which normally is a cone-shaped portion that contains a wick lining the circumference of the internal surface [19]. The control unit controls the water supply into the wick. The cone-shaped part of the HCH is inserted into a heat source. When inspiration occurs, the supply gas from the ventilator flows through the paper media in the cone-shaped portion and additional heat and moisture is added to the inspired gas from the wick surface. However, with expiration, the additional heat and moisture is absorbed by the wick surface to reload the HCH [19].

It is worth mentioning that for AHMEs the temperature setting of 37°C is unchangeable. Based on the minute ventilation, which is normally set by a clinician, the control unit adjusts the heat source and water

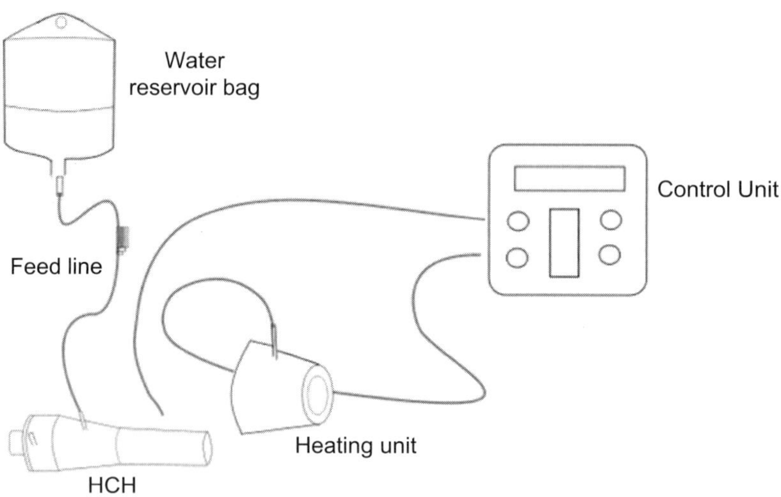

Figure 4-1. Components of an Active Heat and Moisture Exchanger (AHME)

supply to the wick surface. During operation, the HCH, which is part of the AHME, provides moisture of approximately 28 to 31 mg/L. Under a humidifier moisture output setting of 44 mg/L, the heated portion of the AHME is only required to supply 13 to 16 mg/L of moisture to reach the desired value. This type of humidifier is designed to eliminate the problem of condensation in the air delivery tube [18]. The total dead space of an AHME is typically 73 ml. As the AHME undergoes passive operation, it would have the same main disadvantage as a passive humidifier, which is the high dead space that can impact on spontaneously breathing and paralyzed patients [19].

To prevent the side effects of using CPAP, a humidifier is an essential addition to the system. However, it has been shown that the use of a heated humidifier during the initial phase of CPAP treatment does not introduce any significant initial improvement in patient comfort [12].

A humidifier should be used on patients with a dry nose, nasal congestion, or dry throat [12]. It was demonstrated that humidification of inspired air can prevent or reduce dehydration of inspired air during CPAP treatment, particularly in patients complaining of nasal symptoms and suffering from a conditions likely to promote mouth leaks [3]. Humidification can be achieved for the pressurized air in the CPAP system to prevent side effects, but not all systems provide the same amount of humidification.

4.3 MODELING WITH HUMIDIFICATION

The main purpose of this chapter is to analyze the thermal performance of the CPAP machine. The physical laws of thermodynamics and heat transfer will be used to develop governing equations simulating the dynamic system. This will give the dynamic fluctuating outputs of evaporation in the chamber, as well as temperature changes in the delivery tube and mask. The model can also provide steady state outputs. By formulating a model that incorporates the relationship between the inputs and measurable outputs of each individual system element, in terms of air conditions at the mask, the overall performance of the whole system can also be determined.

Thus, it can be used to make comparisons between steady state outputs and breathing-introduced fluctuating outputs. When using a CPAP machine, all the components and water will be at the ambient temperature prior to switching on. When the machine is switched on, the temperatures will move through a transient phase, until a steady state is achieved. The thermodynamic model developed in this section does not account for the warm-up period. The system inputs include ambient air conditions, mask size, pressure, heating element setting, delivery tube heating setting, and the patient's breath load.

Although the CPAP system was explained in Chapter 3, a summary is given here for easy access and clarity. The system consists of an air delivery unit, a humidifier, a heated air delivery tube, a flexible tube and a nasal mask.

The main function of the air delivery unit is to provide the desired air pressure to maintain CPAP at the mask. The heated humidifier receives the air from the air delivery unit, humidifies it by adding water vapor, and then delivers it to the air delivery tube. To prevent condensation in the air delivery tube while the moist air flows toward the nasal mask, a heating wire system is embedded inside the tube wall to maintain the airflow temperature above its dew point. The air is conveyed to the mask via a lighter flexible tube. Dynamic energy balance calculations for each individual component are shown in the sections that follow, and a model is developed for the overall system.

4.4 AIR DELIVERY UNIT

As stated in the previous chapter the main purpose of the air delivery unit is to supply the required range of airflow rates under predetermined pressures. In general the output of the unit is proportional to the input, which gives an ideal zero order element with no delay. The outlet temperature is influenced by the inlet air temperature, operating temperature, and the air delivery unit efficiency. To determine the heated humidifier intake air conditions, it is important to determine the relationship between the intake air temperature and the outlet air temperature under different air mass flow rate settings. For compressible flow through a compressor machine, appreciable changes of fluid density can be expected. For air, changes in density are related to changes in pressure and temperature according to the equation of state. However, in this allocation the change in density is very small and can be neglected.

The first law of thermodynamics for steady flow may be given by [24]:

$$\dot{Q} - \dot{W}_d = \dot{m} \cdot (H_2 - H_1) + \frac{1}{2} \cdot \left(v_2^2 - v_1^2\right) + g \cdot (z_2 - z_1) \qquad (4-2)$$

where $\dot{Q}$ is heat transfer per second, $\dot{W}_d$ work done per second, $\dot{m}$ mass flow rate, H airflow specific enthalpy, v fluid flow velocity and z is elevation relative to some external reference point.

Assuming constant specific heat c_p, the change in enthalpy may be written as:

$$H_2 - H_1 = c_p \cdot (T_2 - T_1) \qquad (4-3)$$

For gases the potential energy term $g \cdot (z_2 - z_1)$ is very small and can be neglected. Assuming the flow processes to be adiabatic ($\dot{Q} = 0$). Thus equation (4-2) can be written as:

$$\dot{W}_d = \dot{m} \cdot \left[\left(H_2 + \frac{1}{2} \cdot v_2^2 \right) + \left(H_1 + \frac{1}{2} \cdot v_1^2 \right) \right] \qquad (4-4)$$

The stagnation enthalpy is defined as:

$$H_T = H + \frac{1}{2} v^2 \qquad (4-5)$$

Using this equation for H_1 and H_2 and then substituting into equation (4-4) results in:

$$\dot{W}_d = \dot{m} \cdot (H_{T_2} - H_{T_1}) \qquad (4-6)$$

The compression process between the inlet and outlet pressure of the compressor, P_1 and P_2, respectively, can be assumed adiabatic with no losses. Thus the process may be assumed isentropic. However, in the actual process, the friction loss increases the input energy (enthalpy) requirement; therefore, the true increase of enthalpy is along line 1-3 of the compression process given in Figure 4-2. The isentropic efficiency of a compressor can be defined as:

$$\eta_i = \frac{isentropic \;\; work}{Actual \;\; work} = \frac{H_{T_2} - H_{T_1}}{H_{T_3} - H_{T_1}} \qquad (4-7)$$

Here, the compressor isentropic efficiency needs to be determined empirically by measuring the input and output temperatures at different compressor pressure settings, P_s. Typical relationships were developed for a compressor used in a CPAP device by Sun [16] and are used here. Using relationships from air table curve fitting techniques, η_i was expressed as:

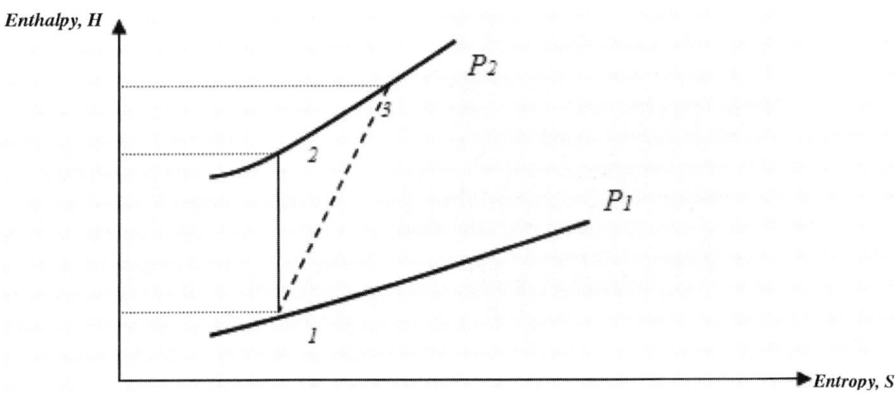

Figure 4-2. Enthalpy/entropy diagram for a compressor

$$\eta_i = 0.4465 \cdot P_s + 25.2 \tag{4-8}$$

and the air delivery unit outlet temperature T_3 was written as:

$$T_3 = \frac{H_{T_3} - 1.0567}{1.0042} \tag{4-9}$$

4.5 HUMIDIFICATION PROCESS

The main function of the humidifier in a CPAP system is to heat and humidify the airflow received from the air delivery unit. Instead of controlling humidity directly, it controls the temperature and humidification as a secondary effect [5]. A typical humidifier chamber is shown in Figure 4-3; the design geometry is aimed at higher vapor-air mixing efficiency (creates turbulent flow and increases airflow time inside the chamber). In this section, the basic chamber heat and mass transfer mathematical model will be developed. The humidifier consists of a reservoir with an aluminum base in contact with a heating system. The chamber heating system consists of the heating element contacting the chamber base to provide heat to the water. The reservoir consists of two parts: the lower part is the water container and the upper part is the air chamber, which allows air to pass over the water surface for humidification purposes.

When the water is heated, the airflow in contact with the water surface will be heated and humidified mainly by water molecule evapora-

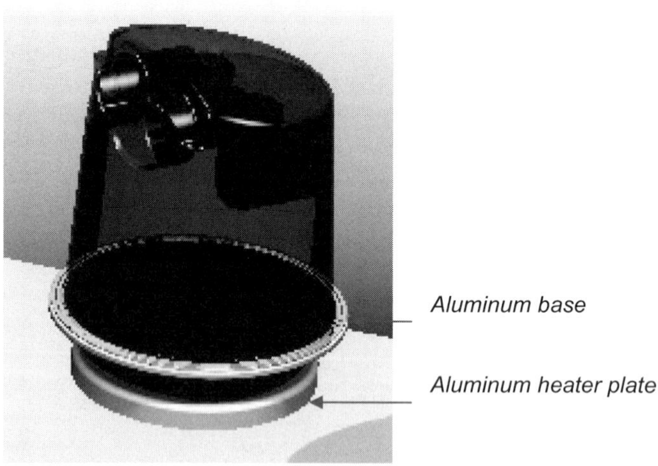

Figure 4-3. Typical humidification chamber [Courtesy of Fisher & Paykel Healthcare Ltd]

tion from the water surface. The CPAP machine is normally designed to control the heating element temperature. The factors influencing water temperature may include heating element temperature setting, ambient air temperature and humidity, pressure setting, airflow rate, and airflow velocity over the water surface as well as flow pattern and flow direction on the surface. The evaporation rate also influences heat taken away from the water, thus influencing water temperature. Chamber geometry, size, structural layout, and material of mask are also related factors. The chamber geometry design is aimed at higher heat and mass (vapor) transfer rate from the water to the airflow. A high Nusselt number and mass convection (evaporation) coefficient are generated by creating turbulent flow, letting the air have longer contact with water and trying to avoid airflow shortcuts from the chamber inlet directly to the outlet.

Figure 4-4 shows the chamber water heat balance. Figure 4-5 shows a flowchart of the heat delivered to the humidifier. Heat flows into the water from the heating element at the humidifier base. There is some heat loss from the rim of the heater plate to the surroundings before heat is delivered to the water. As the water is heated, there are heat losses from the humidifier walls to the surroundings. In the air chamber, the upper part of the humidifier, heat energy is delivered to the air by mass transfer (evaporation) and convection. There are some heat losses from the air to the surroundings.

As explained in previous sections, the main mechanism of the humidification in a CPAP humidifier is mass transfer by evaporation. In

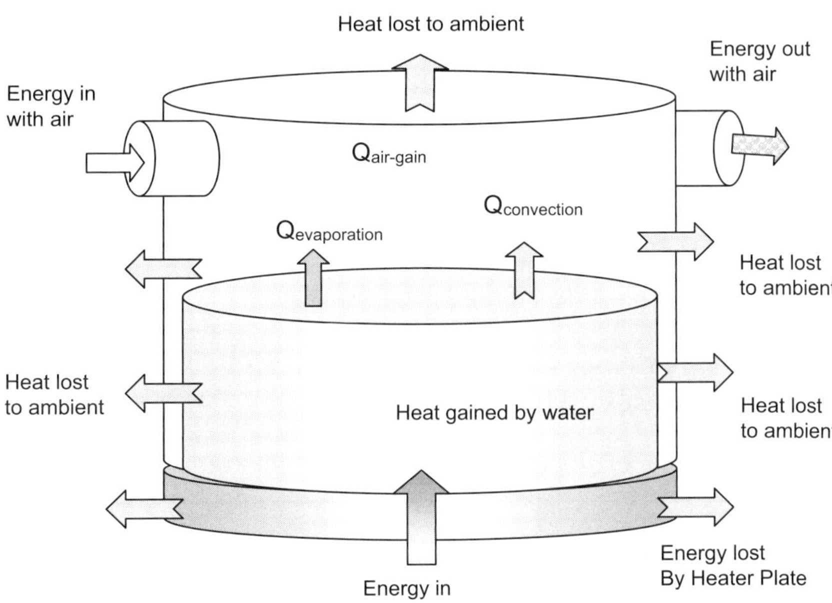

Figure 4-4. Energy balance of a heated humidifier

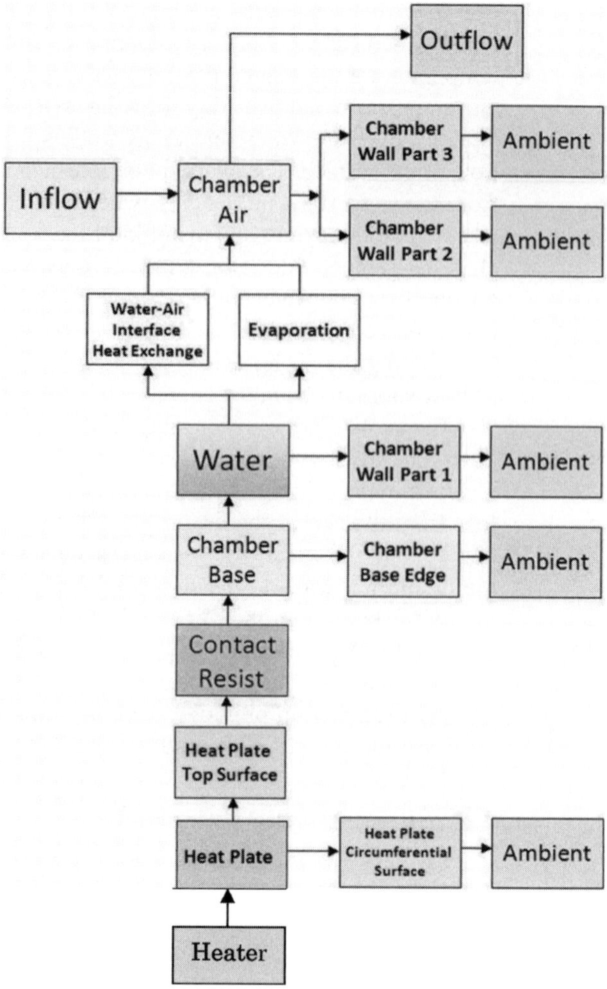

Figure 4-5. Humidifier energy flow

the following sections, we will discuss the mass transfer process first, followed by complete heat transfer analysis of the humidifier.

4.6 MASS TRANSFER

Heated humidification is an air-conditioning process in which water vapor is added to the air stream and there is simultaneous transfer of heat and mass (water vapor) between the air stream and wetted surface, which is the heated reservoir surface. Mass transfer by molecular dif-

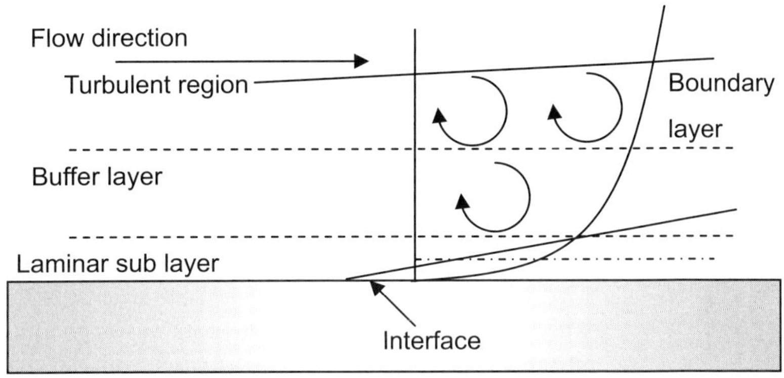

Figure 4-6. Turbulent diffusion boundary layer on a flat surface

fusion or convection is the process of transporting one component of a mixture due to concentration gradients [25]. The driving force for the phase change is the concentration difference. The flow of the commodity is always in the direction of decreasing concentration (from high to low concentration). For evaporation, the driving force is the vapor pressure difference [26]. In a typical humidification chamber, the airflow enters the chamber and flows over the wetted surface before it leaves the chamber.

Consider an air stream in steady turbulent flow over a wetted surface, as shown in Figure 4-6. Assume the liquid-vapor interface is stationary with zero velocity. This creates laminar flow adjacent to the wetted surface. A transition region exists at the buffer layer between the laminar sub layer and the main turbulent stream. In this region the fluid may alternatively be laminar or turbulent. In general, only molecular diffusion can occur within the laminar sub layer. In the buffer layer, both molecular and eddy diffusion, which contribute to the mass transfer, can exist. Eddy diffusion, which is predominant in the turbulent region, is so rapid that it almost equalizes the concentration gradient. The mass transfer rate M_B'' at the interface may be written as [25]:

$$M_B'' = \left(h_m \cdot {}^{M_B}\!/_{R_g} \right) \cdot A_{reservoir} \cdot (P_{Bi} - P_{Bo}) \qquad (4-10)$$

where h_m is the mass transfer coefficient in the airflow and reservoir surface $A_{reservoir}$ interface; M_B is the molecular mass; R_g is universal gas constant; and P_{Bi} and P_{Bo} are the vapor pressures at the chamber airflow and reservoir interface and chamber inlet airflow, respectively. Both M_B and R_g are constants so the relationship can be simplified to:

$$M_B'' = K_m \cdot A_{reservoir} \cdot (P_{Bi} - P_{Bo}) \qquad (4-11)$$

with

$$K_m = h_m \cdot {M_B}/{R_g} \qquad (4-12)$$

where h_m is the mass transfer coefficient, which can be expressed as [27]:

$$h_m = \frac{h_r}{c_{pm}} \qquad (4-13)$$

where h_r is the forced convection heat transfer coefficient; and ***Cpm*** is the specific heat of moist air. ***Cpm*** increases with the chamber air humidity ratio W_a according to:

$$c_{pm} = c_p + W_a \cdot c_{ps} \qquad (4-14)$$

where c_{ps} is the specific heat of the reservoir.

The airflow pattern inside the humidification chamber varies with the discharged airflow from the air delivery unit and h_r. To simplify the mathematical model, K_m can be determined by a simple relationship between airflow velocity and heater plate setting, which can be determined experimentally by measuring the absolute humidity levels of the airflow before and after humidification [16]. The mass transfer equation for a typical humidifier can then be expressed as [25]:

$$M_B'' = C_m \cdot V \cdot A_{reservoir} \cdot (P_{Bi} - P_{Bo}) \qquad (4-15)$$

The chamber airflow vapor pressure depends on its inlet saturation pressure of water at airflow temperature, P_{gai}, and relative humidity, ϕ_i. The chamber airflow vapor pressure can then be expressed as:

$$P_{Bo} = \phi_i \cdot P_{gai} \qquad (4-16)$$

The vapor pressure at chamber airflow and reservoir interface P_{Bi} is defined as the saturation pressure at chamber reservoir temperature *Tw*. The air delivery unit raises the airflow temperature, which is mainly due to the low efficiency of the blower. The chamber inlet air relative humidity will always be lower compared with the ambient relative humidity, but the absolute humidity and specific humidity levels will not change as no moisture is being added or removed during the process. The ambient air absolute humidity, *AH*, can be written as [28]:

$$AH = \omega \cdot \rho_{air} \qquad (4-17)$$

where ω and ρ_{air} are the ambient air specific humidity and density. The air specific humidity depends on atmospheric pressure, P_∞, ambient relative humidity, ϕ, and saturation pressure of water at ambient air temperature, P_g. It represents the mass of water vapor in a unit mass of air. The ambient air specific humidity can be calculated by [28]:

$$\omega = \frac{0.622 \cdot \phi \cdot P_g}{P_\infty - \phi \cdot P_g} \qquad (4-18)$$

As the air delivery unit raises the airflow temperature and pressure, it increases the airflow saturation pressure of water, which results in a drop in the relative humidity level. The air delivery unit outlet airflow relative humidity can be calculated by [28]:

$$\phi_i = \frac{\omega \cdot P_s}{(0.622 + \omega) \cdot P_{gai}} \qquad (4-19)$$

Since the connection between the air delivery unit and the chamber is very small, the temperature drop between the air delivery unit outlet and chamber inlet is neglected and the relative humidity remains constant.

4.7 HUMIDIFIER HEAT TRANSFER

The vapor pressure difference is proportional to the water vapor concentration difference (concentration gradient), which is necessary to determine the evaporation rate inside the chamber. The water vapor molecules in the air exert a pressure, which reaches saturation pressure when the air is saturated with water vapor. This pressure depends only on the water temperature. As the water temperature increases, the mean energy of the water molecules increases, which results in more molecules being able to escape from the water surface, thus increasing the saturated vapor pressure. The air chamber part of the humidifier, however, introduces a dynamic effect into the system due to its constant pressure specific heat capacitance.

For organizational purposes, this section is divided into three subsections: Heater Plate, Water Reservoir, and Air Chamber. As the optimum goal is to deliver water vapor to the air in the air chamber, modeling the chamber requires an energy balance (see Figure 4-4). For a period of *dt*, the energy equation can be written as:

$$Energy_{in} - Energy_{out} = Energy_{storage} \qquad (4-20)$$

4.7.1 Heater Plate

Figure 4-7 shows a heater plate where part of the heat is being dissipated to the surroundings. In this section the energy supplied to and

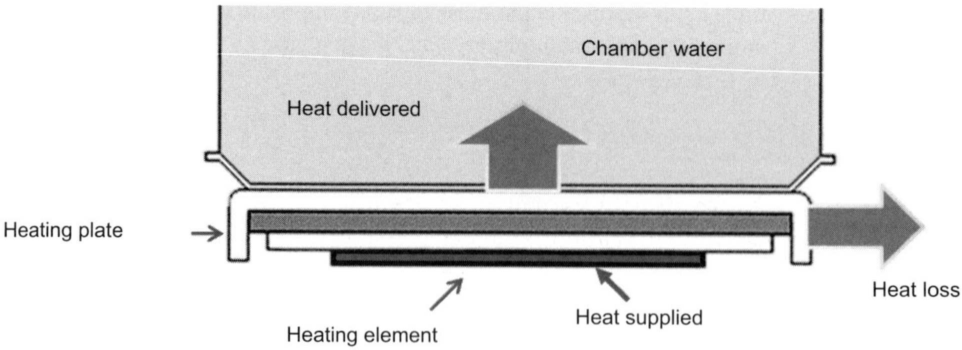

Figure 4-7. Heater plate heat balance

by the heater plate, and the heat supplied at the rim of the plate will be considered.

4.7.1.1 Energy supplied

To determine the humidifier base plate surface temperature, the only energy input for the humidifier is from the heater plate and for a period of *dt*, it can be expressed as:

$$Energy_{in} = \frac{T_e - T_w}{R_{hp}} \cdot dt \qquad (4-21)$$

Where T_e and T_w are the heating element and water temperature, respectively; and R_{hp} is the heater plate overall thermal resistance. To simplify the model, the heater plate thermal capacitance can be neglected without any significant effect on the dynamic behavior of the model.

Heater plates may be typically constructed from a composite of material layers that may include a metal surface plate, a ceramic substrate, and conductive tape. If the material properties are known, the overall thermal resistance of the heater plate can be calculated. However, if there is a lack of data, an experimental approach can be used by setting the heater plate heating elements at a desired temperature, T_e, with thermocouples fitted to the upper surface of the chamber base to measure the chamber base temperature, T_{CB}. Knowing the power input, a system thermal resistance R_{sys} can be determined from:

$$Energy_{in} = \frac{T_e - T_{CB}}{R_{sys}} \qquad (4-22)$$

4.7.1.2 Heat delivered

To determine the humidifier baseplate temperature, attention is directed to the elements of energy loss in the humidifier baseplate. The convection heat transfer coefficient is a function of fluid velocity. The water velocity on the surface of the plate is almost zero, therefore the process of heat transfer from the plate to the water will be considered as natural convection. The natural heat convection coefficient, h_{rnc} depends on the surface characteristic length, δ_r fluid thermal conductivity, k_r, and natural convection Nusselt number, Nu_r [29]. This may be written as:

$$h_{rnc} = \frac{k_r}{\delta_r} \cdot Nu_r \tag{4-23}$$

The characteristic length for a hot plate is defined as:

$$\delta_r = \frac{A_{rb}}{P_{cb}} \tag{4-24}$$

where P_{cb} is the perimeter of the chamber aluminum base. The simple empirical correlations for the average Nusselt number in natural convection can be expressed as [26]:

$$Nu = C \cdot Ra^n \tag{4-25}$$

The values of the constants C and n depend on the geometry of the surface and the flow regime, which are characterized by the range of the Rayleigh number, Ra_r. This can be expressed as:

$$Ra_r = Gr_r \cdot Pr_r \tag{4-26}$$

The Rayleigh number is the product of the Grashof number, Gr_r, and Prandtl number, Pr_r. The Grashof number represents the ratio of the buoyancy force to the viscous force acting on the fluid and it can be written as:

$$Gr_r = \frac{g \cdot \beta_r \cdot (T_{CB} - T_w) \cdot \delta_r^3}{v_r^2} \tag{4-27}$$

where g is the gravitational acceleration. Both fluid thermophysical properties of the coefficient of volume expansion, β_r, and kinematic viscosity, v_r, are to be evaluated at the film temperature, T_f, which can be defined as:

$$T_f = \frac{T_s + T_{fd}}{2} \tag{4-28}$$

where T_s is the heat transfer surface temperature; and T_{fd} is the heat transfer fluid temperature.

To show some typical values of these variables, Sun [16] calculated a film temperature based on the heat transfer surface temperature, T_s; in this case it was the temperature of the chamber base and the heat transfer fluid temperature, T_{fd}. An average Rayleigh number of 5.42 × 10^6 was calculated based on the average operating temperatures of the chamber base and reservoir. This Rayleigh number gives the reservoir natural convection Nusselt number, Nu_r, constants of C = 0.59 and n = 1/4. Through calculation, an average overall thermal resistance of 271.1°C /kW from heater plate heating elements to chamber reservoir was determined.

4.7.1.3 Heat losses

It should be noted that the heater plate circumference surface area, Ahp, is exposed to the atmosphere and heat loss occurs when its temperature is higher than the ambient temperature. Newton's law of cooling expresses the heat energy lost from the heater plate to the ambient surroundings. In a period of *dt*, the rate of the energy loss from the heater plate circumferential surface to the environment, Q_{lostHP}, can be determined by:

$$Q_{lostHP} = h_{hpn} \cdot A_{hp} \cdot (T_e - T_\infty) \cdot dt \qquad (4-29)$$

where h_{hpn} is the natural convection coefficient between the chamber wall and ambient air, which can be determined in the same way as for the water section of the humidifier in the next section. The heater plate surface temperature is assumed to be the same as the heating element temperature.

4.7.2 Water Reservoir

The main heat source for this humidifier section is the heat delivered from the heater plate through the baseplate. The reservoir energy outputs include evaporation energy, heat transfer to the airflow above the reservoir surface, and heat convection loss to the ambient surroundings through the chamber wall below the water level (see Figure 4-4).

4.7.2.1 Heat of evaporation

The energy consumption for evaporation depends on the amount of mass that evaporates and the required latent heat of vaporization, hfg, which is temperature dependent. The amount of water vapor that evaporates can be determined by the mass flow rate difference between the humidifier inlet and outlet. In a period of *dt*, the total energy consumption for evaporation can be expressed as:

$$Energy_{evaporation} = (\dot{m}_{ao} \cdot \omega_o - \dot{m}_{ai} \cdot \omega_i) \cdot h_{fg} \cdot dt \qquad (4-30)$$

where $\dot{m}_{ai}$ and $\dot{m}_{ao}$ are the mass flow rate of the air at the chamber inlet and outlet, respectively; and ω_i and ω_o are the chamber inlet and outlet specific humidity, respectively. As the humidifier chambers usually have complex internal geometry, it is difficult to predict the airflow pattern inside the humidifier chamber under different air delivery unit discharged

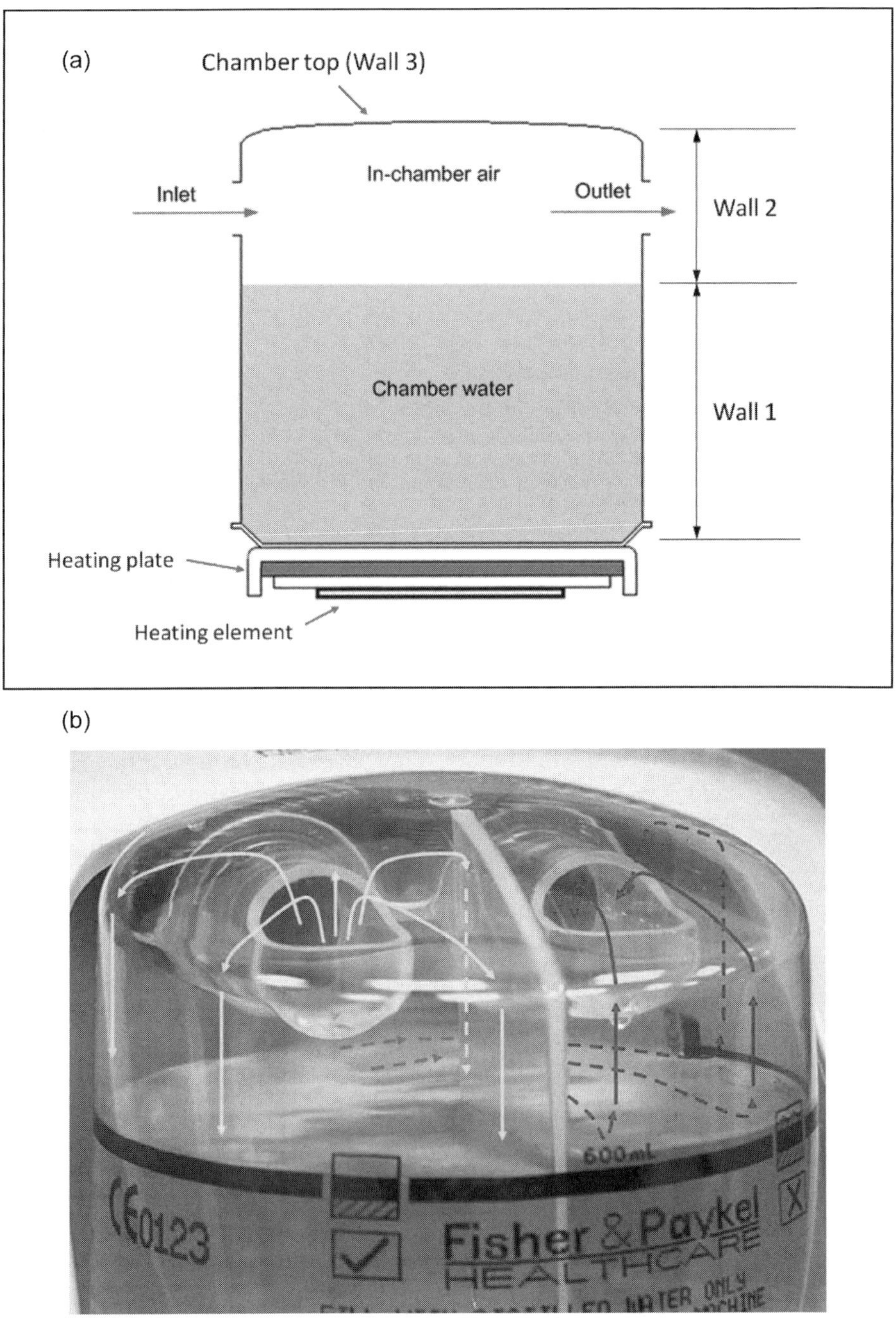

Figure 4-8. **(a)** Humidifier diagram showing water level height **(b)** typical air chamber [Courtesy of Fisher & Paykel Healthcare Ltd]

flow rates. The empirical method is the simplest and most accurate way to determine the forced heat convection coefficient, h_r, between the air and reservoir interface. If we assume that the airflow temperature difference between the inlet and outlet of the humidifier air chamber is caused by the forced heat convection from the reservoir surface only, and the heat gain to the air, $Q_{airgain}$, while it flows through the chamber is due to convection from the hot water surface only, $Q_{convect}$, then

$$Q_{convect} = Q_{airgain} \tag{4-31}$$

with

$$Q_{convect} = h_r \cdot A_{reservoir} \cdot (T_w - T_a) \tag{4-32}$$

and the heat gained by the air

$$Q_{air\ gain} = \dot{m}_{ai} \times C_{pm} \times (T_a - T_{ai}) \tag{4-33}$$

T_{ai} is the chamber inlet temperature; and T_a is the chamber airflow temperature, which is assumed to be the same as the chamber air outlet temperature to keep the model simple.

4.7.2.2 Heat losses through walls

Due to the high water temperature, heat from the humidifier water section dissipates to the ambient surroundings through the reservoir wall (Figure 4-4). The humidifier wall under water level is a vertical cylinder (wall 1), Figure 4-8(a). The reservoir inner wall can be simplified as a vertical flat plate with the inner surface exposed to natural convection with the chamber wall. Since the humidifier, specifically the lower, hotter part, is normally well surrounded by the CPAP case, the radiation dissipation is neglected for simplification. Thus it is assumed that there is only natural convection on the outer surfaces of the chamber. The heat balance at wall 1 may be conducted over a period of dt to get the chamber wall to ambient heat as $Q_{ambient}$:

$$Q_{ambient} = \frac{T_w - T_\infty}{R_{wall1}} \cdot dt \tag{4-34}$$

The thermal resistances to heat flow between the reservoir wall and the ambient include natural convection from reservoir water to walls, thermal conduction through walls, and natural convection from walls to ambient surroundings. The thermal resistance between the reservoir water and wall R_{c1} can be expressed as [26]:

$$R_{c1} = \frac{1}{(2 \cdot \pi \cdot r_{iu} \cdot L_r) \cdot h_{iu}} \tag{4-35}$$

where r_{iu} is the reservoir internal radius under water level. The technique of determining the Grashof and Rayleigh number between reservoir water and wall interface, h_{iu}, is the same as the one for the natural convection coefficient between the chamber base and reservoir. The geometry of a humidifier can be simplified as a vertical cylinder. In this case, the characteristic length, δ_{iu}, for the Grashof number calculation is the height of the water level, L_r. The natural heat convection coefficient can be determined by using equation (4-23).

The heat conduction resistance through the chamber wall, R_{cyl}, depends on its inner and outer radii under water level, r_{iu} and r_{ou} respectively, the height of water level, L_r, and chamber material thermal conductivity, k_{ch} [26].

$$R_{cyl} = \frac{\ln\left(r_{ou} / r_{iu} \right)}{2 \cdot \pi \cdot L_r \cdot k_{ch}} \qquad (4-36)$$

The natural convection resistance from chamber wall surface to ambient, R_{c2}, can be expressed as [26]:

$$R_{c2} = \frac{1}{(2 \cdot \pi \cdot r_{ou} \cdot L_r) \cdot h_{ou}} \qquad (4-37)$$

where h_{ou} is the natural heat convection coefficient between the chamber outer wall surface and the ambient air.

4.7.2.3 Heat balance

The humidifier water reservoir energy storage depends on its mass, m_w, and temperature, T_w. This can be written as:

$$\Delta Energy_{storage} = m_w \cdot c_w \cdot dT_w \qquad (4-38)$$

where c_w is the reservoir specific heat at constant pressure. A reservoir energy balance equation can be obtained by combining all the aforementioned expressions for energy in, out, and storage. In a period of dt, the chamber reservoir energy balance is expressed as:

$$\begin{aligned} \left(\frac{T_e - T_w}{R_{sys}} \right) \cdot dt - (\dot{m}_{ao} \cdot \omega_o - \dot{m}_{ai} \cdot \omega_i) \cdot h_{fg} \cdot dt \\ -[h_r \cdot A_{reservoir} \cdot (T_w - T_a)] \cdot dt \\ -[h_{hp} \cdot A_{hp} \cdot (T_e - T_\infty)] \cdot dt \\ -\left[\frac{T_w - T_\infty}{R_{wall1}} \right] \cdot dt = m_w \cdot c_w \cdot dT_w \end{aligned} \qquad (4-39)$$

Rearranging yields an expression used to model the chamber reservoir temperature as

$$T_w = \frac{1}{\left[m_w \cdot c_w \cdot D + \frac{1}{R_{hp}} + h_r \cdot A_{reservoir} + \frac{1}{R_{wall1}}\right]} \times \left[\frac{T_e}{R_{hp}} - (m_{ao} \cdot \omega_o - m_{ai} \cdot \omega_i) \cdot h_{fg} + h_r \cdot A_{reservoir} \cdot T_a - h_{hp} \cdot A_{hp} \cdot (T_e - T_\infty) + \frac{T_\infty}{R_{wall1}}\right] \quad (4-40)$$

where the operator $D = \frac{d}{dt}$

4.7.3 Air Chamber

In this section the heat delivered to the air and the heat losses from the air chamber to the surrounding are considered. Figure 4-8(a) shows the details of the air chamber boundaries.

4.7.3.1 Heat delivered to air

The chamber airflow temperature greatly influences the chamber reservoir temperature. To simplify the analysis, the airflow temperature drop between the air delivery unit and the chamber inlet is neglected, such that changes in airflow properties can be neglected. The chamber inlet air condition depends on the air delivery unit setting, ambient temperature, and ambient relative humidity. The modeling of airflow temperature inside the humidifier chamber depends mainly on the energy balance. In a period of *dt*, the energy continuity equation can be written as:

$$Energy_{in} - Energy_{out} = Energy_{storage} \quad (4-41)$$

The energy inputs for the chamber air include energy from the chamber inlet airflow and forced heat convection from the hot reservoir surface. In a period of *dt*, the chamber inlet air energy input can be expressed as:

$$Energy_{chamber\ inlet} = \dot{m}_{ai} \cdot c_a \cdot T_{ai} \cdot dt \quad (4-42)$$

where c_a is the air constant pressure specific heat. The amount of energy input by forced heat convection from hot reservoir surface to chamber airflow is exactly the same as the energy lost by forced heat convection from the chamber reservoir. The energy output of the chamber air includes the energy in the chamber outlet airflow and the heat energy lost through the chamber wall to the ambient air. In a period of *dt*, the energy lost by the chamber outlet airflow can be expressed as:

$$Energy_{chamber\ outlet} = \dot{m}_{ao} \cdot c_{pm} \cdot T_a \cdot dt \quad (4-43)$$

4.7.3.2 Wall heat losses

A simplified air chamber geometry and internal airflow pattern is shown in Figure 4-8(a) and Figure 4-8(b), respectively. The simplified top half of the humidifier chamber (chamber internal airflow region) has been separated into two chamber wall parts, No. 2 and No. 3. Wall No. 2 is a vertical tube and No. 3 is a flat circular plate that represents the ceiling of the humidifier chamber. To simplify the airflow, it is assumed that air enters the humidifier chamber and flows over the inner surfaces of the chamber wall No. 2 and No. 3 only once, such that the contact surfaces for wall No. 2, A_{iwall2}, and wall No. 3, A_{iwall3}, are the internal chamber wall surface areas.

In a period of dt, the chamber airflow energy lost to the ambient air through the chamber wall $Q_{wall\text{-}amb}$ can be expressed as:

$$Q_{wall-amb} = \frac{T_a - T_\infty}{R_{wall2}} \cdot dt + \frac{T_a - T_\infty}{R_{wall3}} \cdot dt \qquad (4-44)$$

where R_{wall2} and R_{wall3} are the total thermal resistances of wall No. 2 and No. 3, respectively. The total thermal resistance through the chamber wall from the warm chamber airflow to the ambient air consists of three types: heat convection on the inner and outer surfaces plus heat conduction through the wall itself. The forced heat convection heat transfer resistance between the chamber airflow and chamber wall No. 2 can be defined as:

$$R_{iwall2} = \frac{1}{h_{iwall2} \cdot A_{iwall2}} \qquad (4-45)$$

The forced heat convection coefficient at the chamber inner wall surface, h_{iwall2}, can be expressed as:

$$h_{iwall2} = \frac{k_{ca}}{L_{ca}} \cdot Nu_{ca} \qquad (4-46)$$

where k_{ca} and L_{ca} are the chamber airflow thermal conductivity and height of the chamber airflow region. For forced convection, the Nusselt number, Nu_{ca}, depends on the condition of the airflow that flows above the heat transfer surface. A non-dimensional Reynolds number, Re_{ca}, which describes the chamber airflow condition is defined as:

$$Re_{ca} = \frac{V_{ca} \cdot L_{wall2}}{\nu_{ca}} \qquad (4-47)$$

where V_{ca} and L_{wall2} are the chamber airflow velocity and airflow length, respectively. In this case L_{wall2} is the circumference of the chamber inner wall. For simplicity, the chamber airflow velocity is assumed to be the same as the chamber inlet airflow velocity. The chamber airflow properties, such as kinematic viscosity, v_{ca}, thermal conductivity, k_{ca}, and Prandtl number, Pr_{ca}, can be determined using the chamber airflow film temperature. As mentioned earlier, the chamber airflow is always in a turbulent state within the air delivery unit operating conditions; therefore, the Nusselt number for the entire chamber wall No. 2 inner wall surface is determined by using the Colburn equation [26] as:

$$Nu_{ca} = 0.037 \cdot Re_{ca}^{0.8} \cdot Pr_{ca}^{\frac{1}{3}} \qquad (4-48)$$

With known average chamber airflow heat convection Nusselt and Reynold's numbers, the average forced heat convection coefficient and thermal resistance for chamber wall No. 2 are determined using equations (4-45) and (4-46). It should be noted that chamber wall No. 2 has the same simplified geometry (vertical cylinder) as the chamber wall below water level. Therefore, its thermal conduction resistance can be found by utilizing equation (4-35) with chamber wall No. 2 inner, r_{iwall2}, and outer, r_{iwall2}, radii and the height of the chamber airflow region.

The technique to calculate the thermal natural convection resistance between the chamber wall No. 2 external surface and ambient air is identical to the procedure used to determine the natural convection resistance from the chamber wall under water level to the ambient air. To simplify the analysis, it has been assumed that chamber wall No. 2 and No. 3 are at the same temperature under all operating conditions.

Chamber wall No. 3 has been simplified as a simple circular plate and so the heat convection coefficient, h_{iwall3}, at its inner surface can be expressed as [26]:

$$h_{iwall3} = \frac{k_{ca}}{D_{w3}} \cdot Nu_{w3} \qquad (4-49)$$

where D_{w3} and Nu_{w3} are the chamber wall No. 3 diameter and forced convection Nusselt number. The Reynolds number, Re_{w3} that describes the airflow condition over the inner wall No. 3 surface can be defined as [26]:

$$Re_{w3} = \frac{V_{ca} \cdot D_{w3}}{v_{ca}} \qquad (4-50)$$

Applying the Reynold's number for inner wall No. 3 to equation (4-48) gives its forced heat convection Nusselt number, Nu_{w3}. Utilizing equation (4-49) with Nu_{w3} gives the chamber wall No. 3 forced heat convection coefficient h_{iwall3}. Implementing this with the known surface area, A_{iwall3}, the forced heat convection resistance can be calculated using equation (4-45).

The thermal conduction resistance through chamber wall No. 3 can be determined with known chamber wall No. 3 material thermal conductivity, thickness, and cross-sectional area. The chamber wall No. 3 natural heat convection thermal resistance from the upper surface to ambient air can be calculated using the same procedure used to determine the natural heat convection resistance between the chamber baseplate and reservoir.

The chamber airflow energy storage depends on its mass, m_a, and temperature. It can be written as:

$$\Delta Energy_{storage} = m_a \cdot c_a \cdot dT_a \qquad (4-51)$$

4.7.3.3 Heat balance

An air chamber energy balance equation can be obtained by combining the expressions of energy in, out, and storage. In a period of *dt*, the chamber reservoir energy balance is expressed as:

$$(\dot{m}_{ai} \cdot c_a \cdot T_{ai}) \cdot dt + [h_c \cdot A \cdot (T_w - T_a)] \cdot dt - (\dot{m}_{ao} \cdot c_a \cdot T_a) \cdot dt - \left(\frac{T_a - T_\infty}{R_{wall2}}\right) \cdot dt - \left(\frac{T_a - T_\infty}{R_{wall3}}\right) = m_a \cdot c_a \cdot dT_a \qquad (4-52)$$

Rearranging equation (4-52) yields the following expression of chamber airflow temperature:

$$T_a = \frac{1}{\dot{m}_a \cdot c_a \cdot s + \left(h_c \cdot A \cdot + \dot{m}_{ao} \cdot c_a + \frac{1}{R_{wall2}} + \frac{1}{R_{wall3}}\right)} \cdot \left(\dot{m}_{ai} \cdot c_a \cdot T_{ai} + h_c \cdot A \cdot T_w + \frac{T_\infty}{R_{wall2}} + \frac{T_\infty}{R_{wall3}}\right) \qquad (4-53)$$

An overall energy balance for the heated humidifier is shown in Figure 4-4. The energy balance of the humidifier provides the chamber airflow water vapor concentration gradient; therefore, the mass transfer rate can be calculated.

Once the amount of water vapor that has been added into the chamber airflow is known, the humidifier output airflow absolute humidity can easily be calculated. The dew point temperature of the chamber outlet airflow can be determined based on its vapor pressure [using equation (4-19)] and dew point temperature relationship. Equation (4-18), with known chamber outlet airflow specific humidity and chamber air pressure, can determine the humidifier chamber outlet airflow vapor pressure.

4.8 HEATED AIR DELIVERY TUBE (HADT)

As the heated moist air flows toward the nasal mask, the heat loss through the delivery tube wall to the ambient surroundings cools down

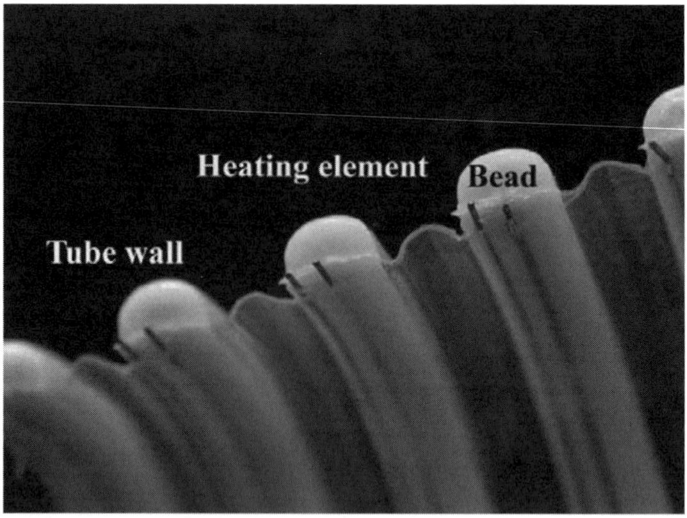

Figure 4-9. Typical heated tube wall [Courtesy of Fisher & Paykel Healthcare Ltd]

the air. Condensation occurs when airflow temperature drops below the dew point temperature and causes the airflow humidity levels to drop. To combat this problem, air delivery tubes that are heated along their lengths have been introduced (see Figure 4-9). The heated air delivery tube (HADT) is usually embedded with a spiral heating element inside the tube wall to maintain the tube wall temperature above the airflow dew point temperature. To simplify the analysis, the thermal contact loss between the heating element and tube wall material is neglected.

The tube heating element efficiency and thermal capacitance are neglected without any significant effect on the dynamic behavior of the model. The thermal resistance of heat conduction through the thin tube wall is ignored for simplicity. The heat transfer through the tube may be modeled as a distributed model approach where a partial differential equation has to be solved, or a simplified lumped approach is used. In this chapter, the latter is used for simplicity. Dividing the tube into 10 lumps, shown in Figure 4-10, accounts for the temperature change experienced along the tube length [16]. This is achieved by using the energy balance

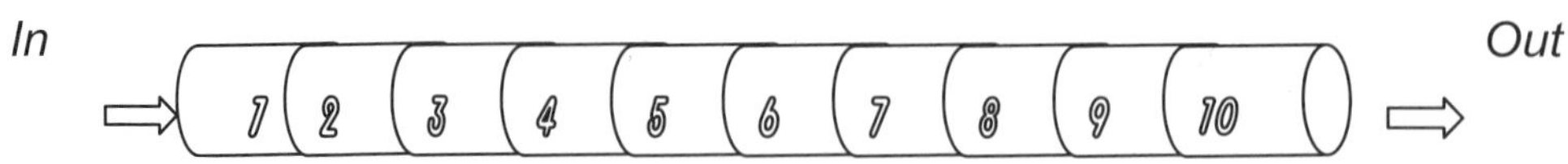

Figure 4-10. Lumped modeling of the HADT

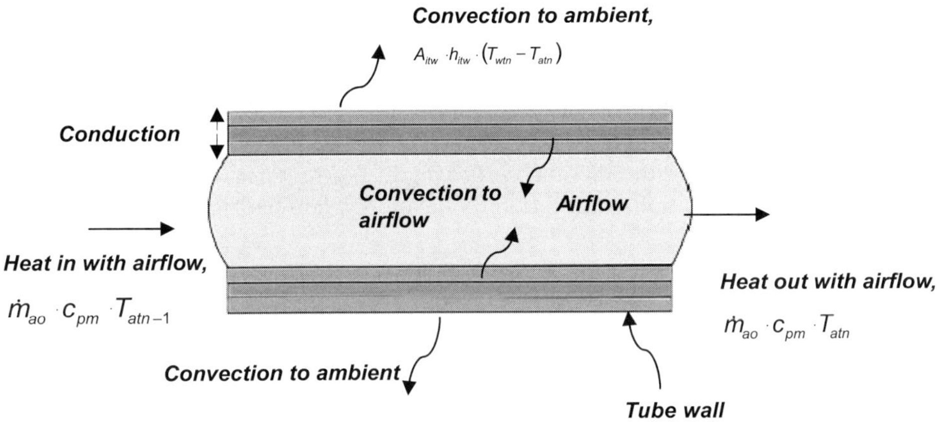

Figure 4-11. Energy balance for each lump of the heated air delivering tube

between the lumped element airflow and wall, shown in Figure 4-11. For the HADT airflow, the axial conduction is relatively small due to the poor conductivity of air and the existence of the "low resistance" heat flow path offered by the fluid transport [30].

Conservation of energy for each lump in a period of dt leads to:

$$Energy_{airflow\ in} + Energy_{wall\ in} - Energy_{airflow\ out} = Energy_{storage\ in\ lump} \quad (4-54)$$

Using Figure 4-11, this can be rewritten as:

$$\begin{aligned}&(\dot{m}_{ao} \cdot c_{pm} \cdot T_{atn-1}) \cdot dt + (h_{itw} \cdot A_{itw} \cdot (T_{wtn} - T_{atn})) \cdot dt \\ &- (\dot{m}_{ao} \cdot c_{pm} \cdot T_{atn}) \cdot dt = m_{ta} \cdot c_{pm} \cdot dT_{atn}\end{aligned} \quad (4-55)$$

Where A_{itw} is tube internal surface area for each lump, h_{itw} tube internal surface forced heat convection coefficient, m_{ta} airflow mass in each lump of the tube, T_{atn-1} hot tube airflow temperature at lump number n-1, T_{atn} hot tube airflow temperature at lump number n and T_{wtn} is hot tube wall temperature at lump number n.

Rearranging equation (4-55) yields an expression used to model the HADT airflow temperature for each lump.

$$\begin{aligned}T_{atn} = &\frac{1}{(m_{ta} \cdot c_{pm} \cdot D + h_{itw} \cdot A_{itw} + \dot{m}_{ao} \cdot c_{pm})} \\ &\times (\dot{m}_{ao} \cdot c_{pm} \cdot T_{atn-1} + h_i \cdot A_i \cdot T_{wtn})\end{aligned} \quad (4-56)$$

The forced heat transfer coefficient at the HADT internal wall surface for each lump depends on the airflow condition and its properties, which can be found based on its film temperature.

For airflow inside a circular pipe, the Reynolds number, Re_{ht}, can be calculated using equation (4-50) with HADT internal diameter D_{ht}. Under typical operating conditions the chamber airflow, and hence the HADT airflow entry condition, will always be turbulent. As the air flows through the HADT, it transforms into fully developed laminar flow and the thermal entry length, L_{ht}, required for the turbulent airflow to transform into fully developed laminar flow can be calculated by [26]:

$$L_{ht} = 0.06 \cdot Re_{ht} \cdot D_{ht} \cdot Pr_{ht} \qquad (4-57)$$

For typical air delivery tubes used in practice, the thermal entry length is approximately 70% of the entire tube length [16]. To simplify the model, the forced heat convection coefficient at the interface of the HADT wall and tube airflow is calculated based on turbulent flow conditions. The heat transfer Nusselt number for the HADT internal wall can be determined using equation (4-49) with the calculated HADT Reynolds number, Re_{ht}, Nu_{ht}, and airflow Prandtl number, Pr_{ht}. An average forced heat convection coefficient can be calculated by:

$$Nu_{ht} = 0.037 \cdot Re_{ht}^{0.8} \cdot Pr_{ht}^{\frac{1}{4}} \qquad (4-58)$$

For the HADT wall temperature, it is reasonable to neglect the radial temperature variation in the tube wall for a thin wall, while the assumption of rectangular airflow velocity and temperature profiles should be quite accurate for turbulent flow conditions. Since the tube wall is thin and there is no intentional heat sink provided to drain off axial heat flow, heat conduction is low [30]. Since the HADT is intentionally designed to be efficient in transferring heat from the heating element to the HADT airflow (a radial heat flow), the axial heat flow is small. Applying conservation of energy to the HADT wall gives:

$$Energy_{heating\ \ element} - Energy_{loss\ \ to\ \ ambient} - Energy_{loss\ \ to\ \ airflow} = Energy_{storage} \qquad (4-59)$$

This can be rewritten as:

$$q_{in} \cdot dt - h_{hto} \cdot A_{hto} \cdot (T_{htwn} - T_{\infty}) \cdot dt - h_{itw} \cdot A_{itw} \cdot (T_{htwn} - T_{atn}) \cdot dt = m_{htw} \cdot c_{htw} \cdot dT_{htwn} \qquad (4-60)$$

where
q_{in} = HADT power input for each lump; h_{hto} = natural heat convection coefficient at HADT outer surface; A_{hto} = HADT outer surface area for each lump; m_{htw} = HADT mass for each lump; and c_{htw} = HADT wall material constant pressure specific heat.

Rearranging equation (4-60) yields the expression used to model the HADT wall temperature for each lump.

$$T_{htwn} = \frac{1}{m_{htw} \cdot c_{htw} \cdot D + h_{itw} \cdot A_{itw} + h_{hto} \cdot A_{hto}} (q_i + h_{hto} \cdot A_{hto} \cdot T_\infty + h_{itw} \cdot A_{itw} \cdot T_{atn}) \qquad (4-61)$$

The amount of heat energy out from the HADT wall to the airflow is exactly the same as the heat energy input for the airflow from the HADT wall. An average natural heat transfer coefficient from the HADT outer surface to ambient air can be calculated using equation (4-49) with the HADT outer diameter, ambient air thermal conductivity, and HADT outer surface Nusselt number, Nu_{hto}. The HADT outer surface can be seen as a horizontal cylinder and the Nusselt number can be written as [26]:

$$Nu_{hto} = \left\{ 0.6 + \frac{0.387 \cdot Ra_{hto}^{1/6}}{(1 + (0.559 / Pr_{hto})^{9/16})^{8/27}} \right\}^2 \qquad (4-62)$$

where Ra_{hto} is the tube outer surface natural convection Rayleigh number and Pr_{hto} is the Prandtl number.

4.9 INTERFACE

The patient interface serves to deliver the airflow to the patient. For a typical nCPAP system, its interface includes a flexible tube and a nasal mask (see Figure 4-12). The modeling for the two components follows.

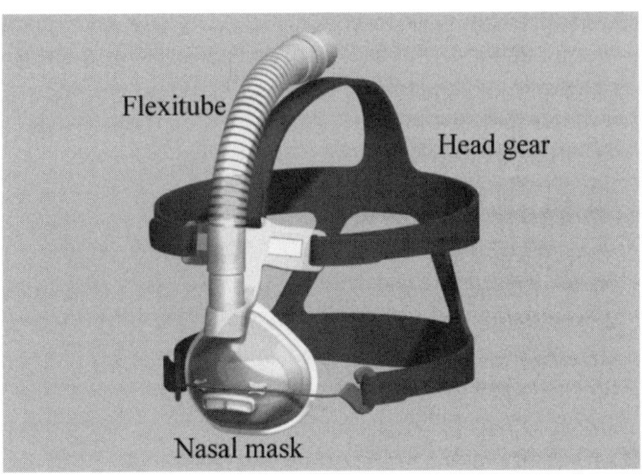

Figure 4-12. nCPAP interface [Courtesy of Fisher & Paykel Healthcare Ltd]

4.9.1 Flexible Tube

The main purpose of this tube is to connect the HADT to the nasal mask (see Figure 4-12). Since it is typically not very long (in the order of 10 to 20 cm), it has been divided into two lumps to increase the accuracy of the model to simulate the temperature change along the tube length. A procedure similar to that used for the HADT is used to evaluate the thermal characteristic of this tube. For simplicity, the thermal resistance of heat conduction through the tube wall is ignored. The energy balance of airflow in the tube is shown in Figure 4-13.

Applying conservation of energy to the airflow in the tube gives:

$$Energy_{in\ \ with\ \ airflow} - Energy_{forced\ \ convection\ \ out} - Energy_{out\ \ with\ \ airflow} = Energy_{storage\ \ each\ \ lump} \qquad (4-63)$$

In a period of dt, the flexible tube airflow thermal energy continuity equation can be written as:

$$\dot{m}_{ao} \cdot c_{pm} \cdot T_{ftn-1} \cdot dt - h_{fti} \cdot A_{fti} \cdot (T_{ftn} - T_{ftwn}) \cdot dt - \dot{m}_{ao} \cdot c_{pm} \cdot T_{ftn} \cdot dt = m_{ft} \cdot c_{pm} \cdot dT_{ftn} \qquad (4-64)$$

Where A_{fti} is the internal wall surface for each lump, h_{fti} the forced heat convection coefficient, m_{ft} the airflow mass in each lump, T_{ftn} the airflow temperature at lump number n, T_{ftn-1} the airflow temperature at lump number n-1, and T_{ftwn} is the wall temperature at lump number n.

Rearranging equation (4-64) yields an expression used to model the airflow temperature in each lump.

$$T_{ftn} = \frac{1}{(m_{ft} \cdot c_{pm} \cdot D + h_{fti} \cdot A_{fti} + \dot{m}_{ao} \cdot c_{pm})} \cdot (\dot{m}_{ao} \cdot c_{pm} \cdot T_{ftn-1} + h_{fti} \cdot A_{fti} \cdot T_{ftwn}) \qquad (4-65)$$

The calculations of forced and natural heat transfer coefficients at the internal and external tube wall surfaces are identical to the HADT wall. To determine the flexible tube wall temperature, the energy balance in a period of dt leads to

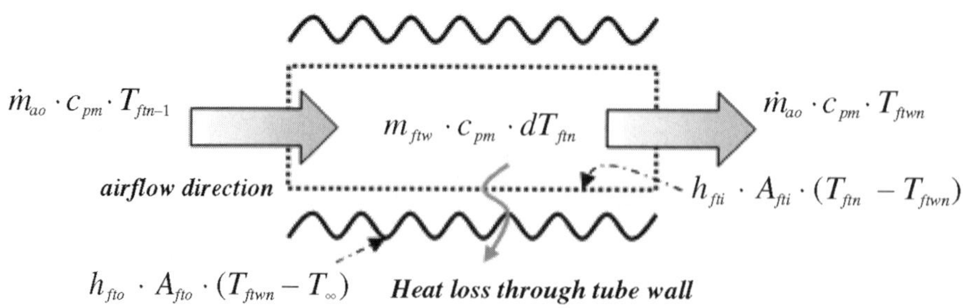

Figure 4-13. Energy balance of a flexible tube

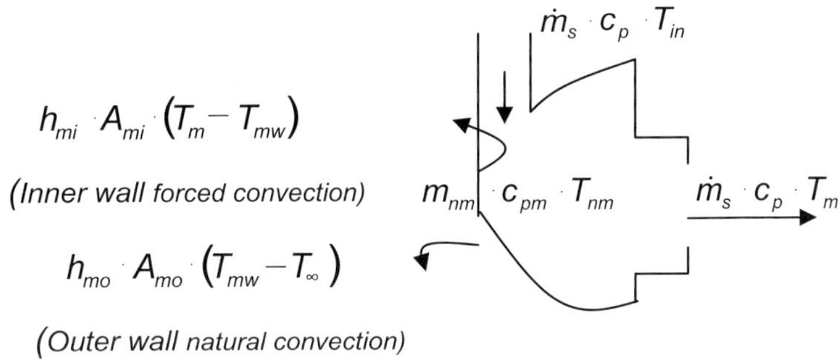

Figure 4-14. Nasal mask airflow energy balance

$$h_{fti} \cdot A_{fti} \cdot (T_{ftn} - T_{ftwn}) \cdot dt - h_{fto} \cdot A_{fti} \cdot (T_{ftwn} - T_{\infty}) \cdot dt = m_{ftw} \cdot c_{ftw} \cdot dT_{ftwn} \qquad (4-66)$$

where A_{fto} the outer surface area for each lump, h_{fto} the outer surface natural heat transfer coefficient, m_{ftw} the mass for each lump and c_{ftn} is the material specific heat at constant pressure.

Rearranging equation (4-66) yields the following expression for the flexible tube wall temperature.

$$T_{ftwn} = \frac{1}{(m_{ftw} \cdot c_{ftw} \cdot D + h_{fti} \cdot A_{fti} + h_{fto} \cdot A_{fto})} \cdot (h_{fti} \cdot A_{fti} \cdot T_{ftn} + h_{fto} \cdot A_{fto} \cdot T_{\infty}) \qquad (4-67)$$

4.9.2 Nasal Mask

The nCPAP airflow is delivered to an OSA patient via a nasal mask and some of it exits through the small vents. The ventilation holes on the nasal mask ensure that fresh air is always available for the patient. For the mask control volume, Figure 4-14, the main input is the air supplied to the mask through the air delivery tube. Minor

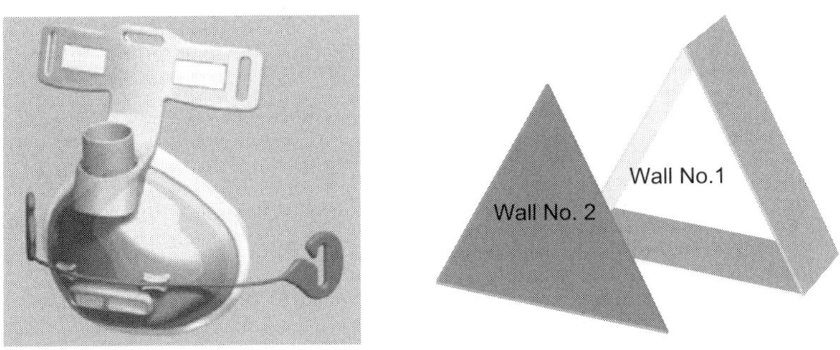

Figure 4-15. Simplified nasal mask geometry

pressure and airflow fluctuations within the nasal mask caused by breathing are ignored, as the pressure fluctuation is always within ±5% of unit positive pressure setting in these types of devices. A bias flow orifice is used to produce the desired mean operating nasal mask air mass flow rates and positive pressures under different air delivery unit settings.

The bias flow condition, instead of "real life" values, is used here for ease of calculation. Patient inhalation absolute humidity level is approximately the same as the nasal mask supply airflow (from the CPAP unit) under the mean air volume flow conditions (bias flow) [17]. A lung simulator, which is capable of providing the proper breathing airflow humidity, temperature, and flow output, could be utilized for more accurate results if desired.

The nasal mask geometry has been simplified as a simple triangular shape and separated into two parts, as shown in Figure 4-15. The airflow pattern inside the nasal mask has been simplified, and the assumption made that nasal mask airflow would flow over the mask internal surfaces only once.

Using the energy balance equation for the airflow across the nasal mask in a period of dt leads to:

$$\dot{m}_{ao} \cdot c_{pm} \cdot T_{in} \cdot dt - h_{im1} \cdot A_{im1} \cdot (T_m - T_{mw}) \cdot dt - h_{im2} \cdot A_{im2} \cdot (T_m - T_{mw}) \cdot dt - \dot{m}_{ao} \cdot c_{pm} \cdot T_m \cdot dt$$
$$= m_{nm} \cdot c_{pm} \cdot dT_m \tag{4-68}$$

where A_{mi1} is the nasal mask wall number 1 internal surface area, A_{mi2} the nasal mask wall number 2 internal surface area, h_{mi1} the nasal mask wall number 1 internal surface forced heat convection coefficient, h_{mi2} the nasal mask wall number 2 internal surface forced heat convection coefficient, m_{nm} the nasal mask airflow mass, T_{ft2} the flexible tube lump No. 2 airflow temperature, T_m the nasal mask air temperature and T_{mw} is the nasal mask wall temperature.

Rearranging equation (4-68) yields an expression for nasal mask airflow temperature to be used in the model.

$$T_m = \frac{1}{m_{mn} \cdot c_{pm} \cdot D + \dot{m}_{ao} \cdot c_{pm} + h_{im1} \cdot A_{im1} + h_{im2} \cdot A_{im2}} \times \left[\dot{m}_{ao} \cdot c_{pm} \cdot T_{ft2} + (h_{im1} \cdot A_{im1} + h_{im2} \cdot A_{im2}) \cdot T_{mw}\right] \tag{4-69}$$

With known mask airflow temperature, backpressure (air delivery unit setting), and specific humidity (identical to the chamber outlet with the assumption of no condensation), the nCPAP unit supplied airflow relative humidity can be calculated based on equation (4-18).

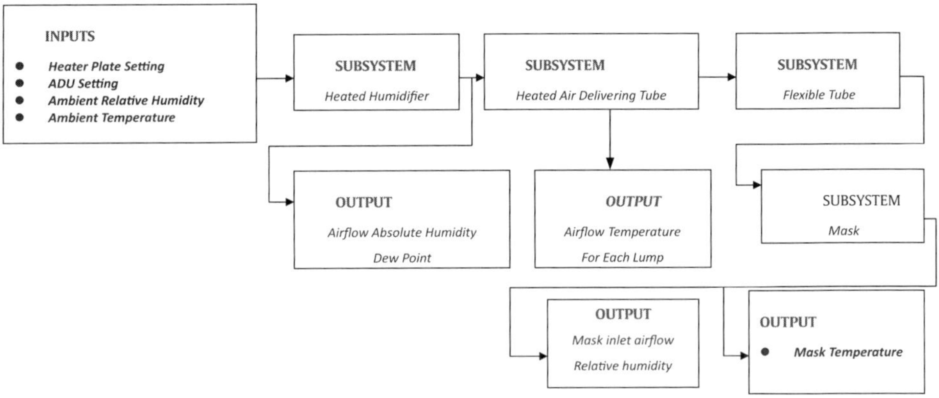

Figure 4-16. Block diagram of nCPAP system

The technique to determine the forced convection coefficients for mask wall Nos. 2 and 3 is identical to the chamber airflow.

The chamber wall temperature energy balance in a period of dt can be expressed as:

$$h_{mi1} \cdot A_{mi1} \cdot (T_{mn} - T_{mw}) \cdot dt + h_{mi2} \cdot A_{mi2} \cdot (T_{mn} - T_{mw}) \cdot dt - h_{mo1} \cdot (T_{mw} \cdot T_{\infty}) \cdot dt - h_{mo2} \cdot A_{mo2} \cdot (T_{mw} - T_{\infty}) \cdot dt = m_{mw} \cdot c_{mw} \cdot dT_{mw} \quad (4-70)$$

where c_{mw} is the nasal mask material specific heat at constant pressure. Rearranging equation (4-70) yields an expression for the nasal mask wall temperature:

$$T_{mw} = \frac{1}{(m_{mw} \cdot c_{mw} \cdot D + h_{mi1} \cdot A_{mi1} + h_{mi2} \cdot A_{mi2} + h_{mo1} \cdot A_{mo1} + h_{mo2} \cdot A_{mo2})} \times [(h_{mi1} \cdot A_{mi1} + h_{mi2} \cdot A_{mi2}) \cdot T_{mf} + (h_{mo1} \cdot A_{mo1} + h_{mo2} \cdot A_{mo2}) \cdot T_{amb}] \quad (4-71)$$

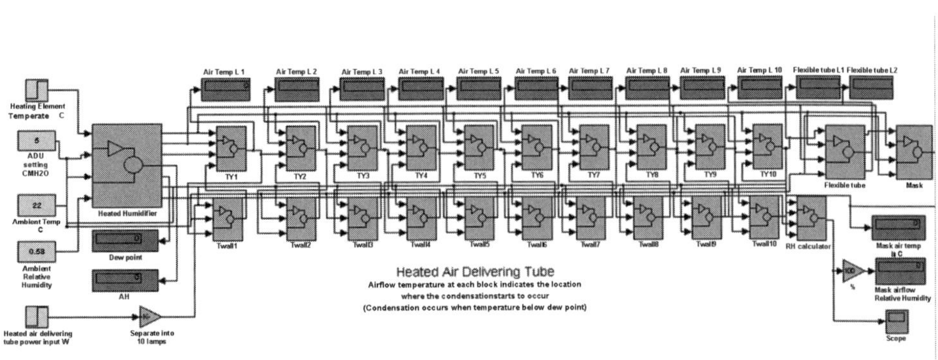

Figure 4-17. Overall nasal CPAP system

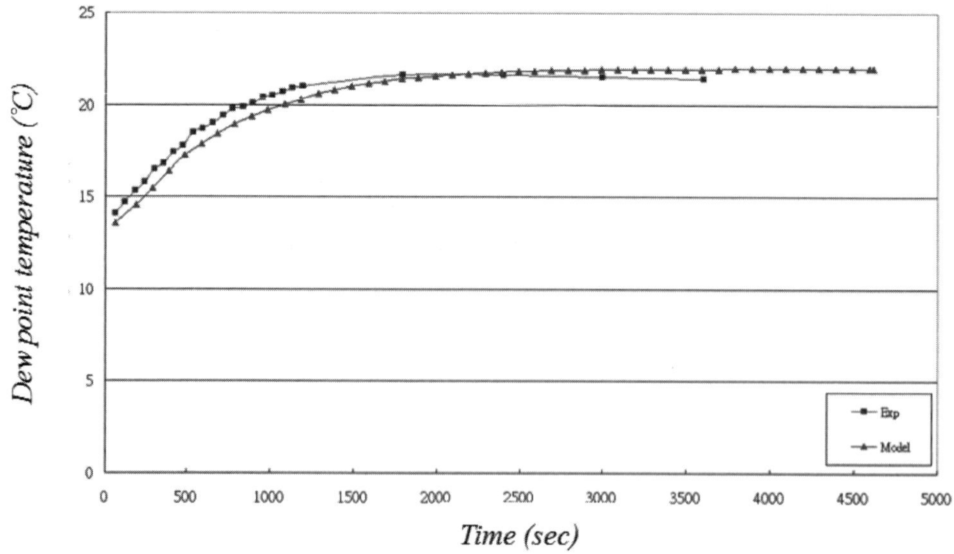

Figure 4-18. Model prediction and experimental results for nasal mask airflow dew point dynamic response under heater plate setting of 45°C

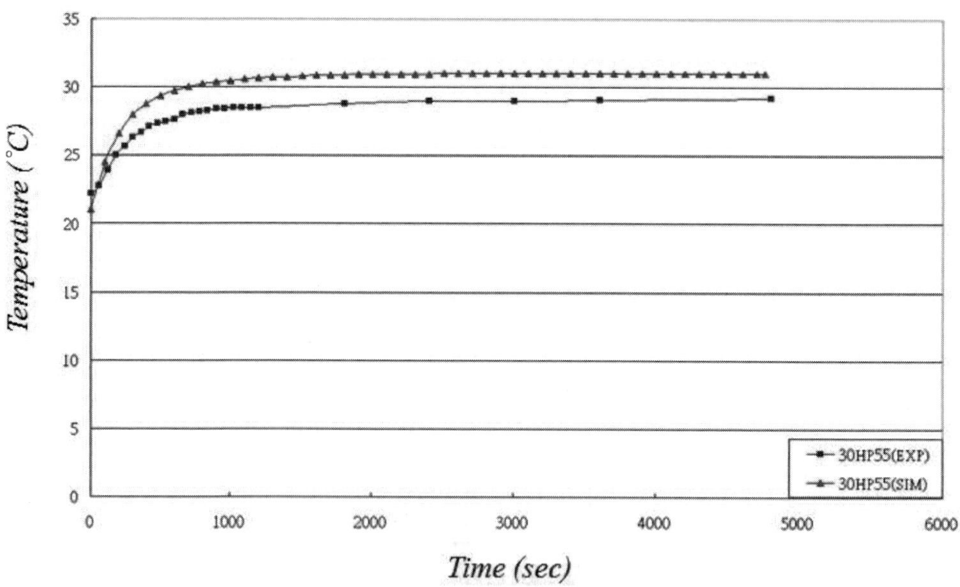

Figure 4-19. Model prediction and experimental results for nasal mask airflow temperature dynamic response

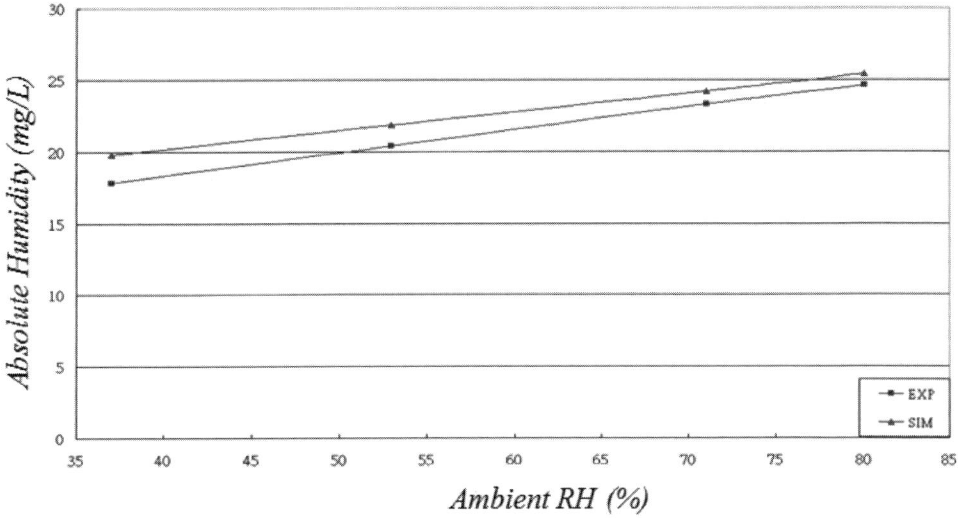

Figure 4-20. Model prediction and experimental results for nasal mask airflow absolute humidity levels under different ambient relative humidity levels

4.10 SIMULINK™ MODEL

The overall functional block diagram of the complete system is shown in Figure 4-16 and its appearance in the Simulink™ is shown in Figure 4-17. Experiments conducted by Sun [16] on a complete nCPAP setup show good congruence with simulations. Since ambient relative humidity and temperature changes are ignored in the simulation, some deviation from experimental results is evident.

A sample comparison of simulation and experimental results for nasal mask airflow dew point under a flow rate of 30 l/min with a heater plate setting of 45°C is shown in Figure 4-18. The simulation error is attributed to overfilling of the humidifier chamber in the experiments, thus increasing the reservoir heat storage and raising its transfer function time constant.

Figure 4-19 shows a comparison of nasal mask supply airflow temperature simulation and experimental results under a constant airflow of 30 l/min, heater plate setting of 55°C, and an HADT power input of 15 W.

The steady state simulation and experimental results of nasal mask supply airflow absolute humidity levels under various ambient relative humidity levels is shown in Figure 4-20, where it is evident that the simulation is able to produce reasonably accurate predictions for unit supply airflow humidity level under various levels of ambient relative humidity.

4.11 CLOSURE

This chapter highlights the need for humidification in CPAP therapy. The different types of humidifiers that are used in practice are discussed. The humidification process in a typical CPAP system is modeled in detail, and comparisons of model and experiments are given at the end of the chapter.

REFERENCES

[1] Randerath, W.J., Meier, J., Genger, H., Domanski, U., Ruhle, K-H., Efficiency of Cold Passover and Heated Humidification Under Continuous Positive Airway Pressure. *Eur Respir J*, 2002. **20**: p. 183–86.

[2] Miyao, H., Miyasaka, K., Hirokawa, T., and Kawazoe, T., Consideration of the International Standard for Airway Humidification Using Simulated Secretions in an Artificial Airway. *Respir Care*, 1996. **41**(1): p. 43–49.

[3] Martins De Araújo, M.T., Vieira, S.B., Vasquez, E.C., and Fleury B., Heated Humidification or Face Mask to Prevent Upper Airway Dryness During Continuous Positive Airway Pressure Therapy. *Chest*, 2000. **117**(1): p. 142–47.

[4] Schulze, A., Respiratory Gas Conditioning in Infants With an Artificial Airway. *Semin Neonatol*, 2002. **7**(5): p. 369–77.

[5] Carter, B.G., Whittington, N., Hochmann, M., and Osborne, A., The Effect of Gas Inlet Temperatures on Heated Humifider Performance. *J Aerosol Med*, 2002. **15**(1): p. 7–13.

[6] Wilkes, A.R., Humidification: Its Importance and Delivery. *BJA CEPD Reviews*, 2001. **1**(2): p. 40–43.

[7] Fujino, Y., Uchiyama, A., Miyoshi, E., Mashimo, T., and Nishimura, M., Inspiratory Gas Temperature in the Endotracheal Tube When Ventilated With a Heated Humidifier. *Critical Care*, 2003. **7**(Suppl 2): p. P158.

[8] Parra, O., Klamburg, J., Xirgu, J., Abad, J., Sala, H., Tomasa, A., and Morera, J., Hygroscopic Condenser Humidifier as a Solution to Nasal Dryness due to Nasal CPAP Treatment for Obstructive Sleep Apnea Syndrome. *Sleep*, 1991. **14**(2): p. 166–68.

[9] Engleman, H.M., Asgari-Jirhandeh, N., McLeod, A.L., Ramsay, C.F., Deary, I.J., and Douglas, N.J., Self-reported Use of CPAP and Benefits of CPAP Therapy: A Patient Survey. *Chest*, 1996. **109**(6): p. 1470–76.

[10] Mortimore, I.L., Whittle, A.T. and Douglas, N.J., Comparison of Nose and Face Mask CPAP Therapy for Sleep Apnoea. *Thorax*, 1998. **53**(4): p. 290–92.

[11] Nilius, G., Effects of Humidification on Nasal Symptoms and Compliance in Sleep Apnea Patients Using Continuous Positive Airway Pressure. *Chest*, 1999. **116**: p. 403–08.

[12] Wiest, G.H., Harsch, I.A., Fuchs, F.S., Kitzbichler, S., Bogner, K., Brueckl, W.M., Hahn, E.G., and Ficker, J.H., Initiation of CPAP Therapy for OSA: Does Prophylactic Humidification During CPAP Pressure Titration Improve Initial Patient Acceptance and Comfort? *Respiration*, 2002. **69**(5): p. 406–12.

[13] Hattori, C., Nishimura, T., Kawakatsu, K., Hayakawa, M., and Suzuki, K., Comparison of Surgery and Nasal Continuous Positive Airway Pressure Treatment for Obstructive Sleep Apnea Syndrome. *Acta Otolaryngol Suppl*, 2003. **550**: p. 46–50.

[14] Nishida, T., Nishimura, M., Fujino, Y., and Mashimo, T., Performance of Heated Humidifiers With a Heated Wire According to Ventilatory Settings. *J of Aerosol Med*, 2001. **14**(1): p. 43–51.

[15] Carter, B.G., Kemp, T., Mynard, J., Hochmann, M., and Osborne, A., Compensating for the Effect of Inlet Gas Temperature on Heated Humidifier Performance. *Anaesth Intensive Care*, 2003. **31**(1): p. 54–57.

[16] Sun, Y.-C., CPAP System Modelling (Humidification Process), Master of Engineering thesis, 2004. Auckland University of Technology, Auckland. p. 190.

[17] Huddart, B.J., Mackie, S.R., and White, C.K., Humidification System, U.S.o.A.P.a.T. Office, Editor, 2007. Fisher & Paykel Healthcare.

[18] Larsson, A., Gustafsson, A., and Svanborg, L., A New Device for 100 Percent Humidification of Inspired Air. *Critical Care*, 2000. **4**(1): p. 54–60.

[19] Branson, R.D., Campbell, R., Johannigmam, J., Ottaway, M., Davis, K. Jr., Luchette, F.A., and Frame, S., Comparison of Conventional Heated Humidification With a New Active Hygroscopic Heat and Moisture Exchanger in Mechanically Ventilated Patients. *Respir Care*, 1999. **44**(8): p. 912–917.

[20] Campbell, R.S., Davis, K. Jr., Johannigman, J.A., and Branson, R.D., The Effects of Passive Humidifier Dead Space on Respiratory Variables in Paralyzed and Spontaneously Breathing Patients. *Respir Care*, 2000. **45**(3): p. 306–12.

[21] Sullivan, C.E., Issa, F.G., Berthon-Jones, M., and Eves, L., Reversal of Obstructive Sleep Apnoea by Continuous Positive Airway Pressure Applied Through the Nares. *Lancet*, 1981. **18**(1): p. 862–65.

[22] Massie, C.A., Hart, R.W., Peralez, K., and Richards, G.N., Effects of Humidification on Nasal Symptoms and Compliance in Sleep Apnea Patients Using Continuous Positive Airway Pressure. *Chest*, 1999 **116**(2): p. 403–08.

[23] Pelosi, P., et al., Relationship Between Absolute humidity of Inspired and Expired Gases With an Active Humidifier. *Critical Care*, 2003. **7**(Suppl 2): p. P155.

[24] Douglas, J.F., Gasiorek, J.M., and Swaffield, J.A., *Fluid Mechanics*, 3rd Ed., 1998. Longman Group, London.

[25] Owen, M.S., Ed., Ashrae Handbook. Vol. Fundamentals, 1981. American Society of Heat, Refrigerating and Air-conditioning Engineers, Atlanta.

[26] Cengel, Y.A. and Turner, R.H., *Fundamentals of Thermal-Fluid Sciences*, 2001. McGraw-Hill, U.S.

[27] Stoecker, W.F. and Jones, J.W., *Refrigeration and Air-Conditioning*, 1982. McGraw-Hill.

[28] Cengel, Y.A. and Boles, M.A., *Thermodynamics: An Engineering Approach*, 3rd Ed., 1998. McGraw-Hill.

[29] Holman, J.P., *Heat Transfer*. SI Metric Ed., 1989. McGraw-Hill.

[30] Doebelin, E.O., *System Modelling and Response, Theoretical and Experimental Approaches* 1st Ed., 1980. John Wiley & Sons, New York.

Chapter 5

CONTROL SYSTEMS FOR CPAP

This chapter focuses on the development of automatic and dynamic control schemes to maintain a constant pressure in Continuous Positive Airway Pressure (CPAP) masks. A control system using a pressure-regulating valve is used as an example throughout this chapter. It demonstrates how lumped parameter modeling can be used to identify time delays and select effective compensation schemes. In this chapter, a feed forward compensation scheme is designed to tackle a time delay problem. The scheme includes adding additional electronic components between the system and the controller. The system control model of a typical CPAP device is developed in Simulink™ in the Matlab™ environment.

5.1 AVAILABLE CONTROL SCHEMES

This section gives an overview of some of the available control techniques used for CPAP devices. The International Organization for Standardization (ISO) is a worldwide federation of national standard bodies. A maximum pressure limitation [1] for CPAP and self-adjusting sleep apnea breathing therapy devices is given in the International Standard ISO 17510-1 Sleep Apnea Breathing Therapy. It states that the maximum achievable pressure at the patient connection port shall not exceed 2 kPa (20 cm H_2O) under normal use and 3 kPa (30 cm H_2O) under single fault condition. The said standard does not mention the allowable mask pressure fluctuation for a breathing cycle or under a fixed pressure setting. Therefore, in this chapter it is assumed that a pressure swing of ± 0.5 cm H_2O is acceptable in the mask.

Currently most of the available CPAP machines use an open loop control scheme as shown in Figure 5-1. In this scheme the CPAP machine has a fixed input mask pressure setting and the mask pressure is

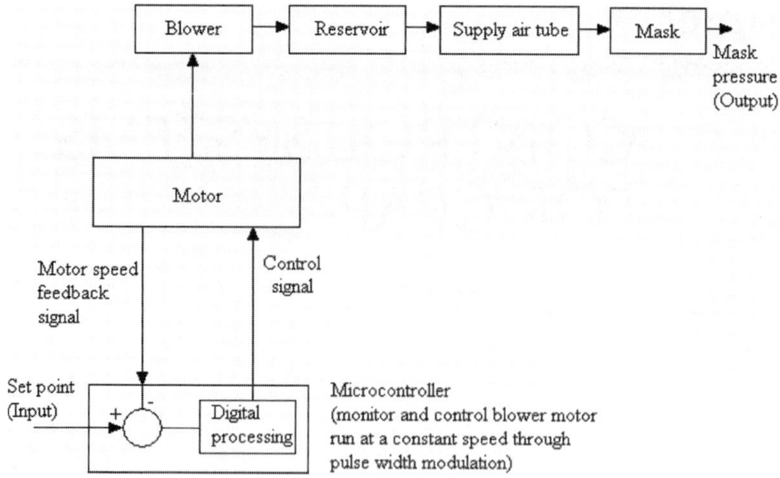

Figure 5-1. Current CPAP control scheme

a function of the variation of the airflow process. Currently most CPAP machines are controlled by a micro-controller. The latter is programmed with software to control the motor, which normally runs at a constant speed. The blower outlet pressure mainly relies on the characteristics of the fan to provide constant pressure as the flow varies due to the patient's breathing action. This system lacks control action to compensate for breath variation during normal circumstance or abnormal activity, such as sneezing, coughing, snoring, etc. Thus a new system must be developed to meet these requirements.

Recent work in the treatment of sleep apnea has included the use of CPAP to maintain the airway of the patient in a continuously open state during sleep. In principle, as the air is delivered through the delivery tube to the mask, an appropriate control scheme is proposed. Some of the available automatic control systems to control the pressure in the mask are summarized below:

A sealed mask is designed to sit over the patient's nose with a pressure release valve to release the air from the mask when it reaches a prescribed pressure level. United States patent number US4655213 [2].

A control method with a feedback mask pressure signal to control the speed of a blower motor to maintain a constant pressure mask is used. The system comprises a differential pressure sensor installed at the mask that sends a pressure signal to a microprocessor, which then sends the signal to an electronic speed control unit to control the blower speed. United States patent number US2002100477 [3].

A control method using a pressure sensor to monitor a flow control valve to maintain a constant mask pressure is used. The system consists of a pressure sensor, a controller, and a flow control valve. As the delivery tube supplies the air, a flow sensor is installed in the mask to measure the pressure. When the pressure changes from a preset value, a signal is sent to the controller, which actuates the flow control valve in accordance with a predesigned control scheme. United States patent number US2002078958 [4].

United States patent number US2002096173 [5] discloses a control method using a pressure transducer to control a gas supply pump to maintain a constant mask pressure. A nasal mask is connected to a gas supply pump via a supply tube. A pressure transducer at the mask is used to measure the mask pressure at the patient's nose. Its output electrical signal is to a servo-controller, which regulates the gas supply pump.

European patent number EP0920845 [6] discloses a control method using a pressure transducer and a differential transducer to feed back the mask pressure and airflow signal to control a blower motor. The control system consists of placing a flow resistive element sensor in the delivery tube between the blower and the mask. This sensor is connected to a pressure differential transducer and a separate pressure transducer. The output signal of the first represents an airflow signal, while that of the second represents a mask pressure signal. Compensations were made for the two signals to account for the delivery tube and other losses. The pressure signal is fed back to a motor servo unit to fine-tune the required mask pressure. Both signals are converted to a digital signal through an analogue to digital converter. The digital signal is then passed through a microprocessor to calculate the set point of the mask pressure. This digital mask pressure set point signal will be converted to an electrical signal through a digital-to-analogue converter to control the motor servo unit.

The first method [2] is an open loop that depends on the pressure release valve to release the excess pressure of the system to maintain the mask pressure constant. The system has several disadvantages. The arrangement is simple and the mask pressure mainly depends on the actual valve release pressure, with no control when the mask pressure is below the valve release setting. Also, the mechanically operated valve may produce annoying sound levels when it releases the excess pressure. In addition, the mask is heavy and bulky due to the installed valve, which may result in patient discomfort. The other methods of control [3-6] use closed loop and micro-controller digital control. They collect and process the mask pressure signal. The processed signal is then used to control the air blower or actuate the valve to adjust the flow of gas through the supply tube to maintain the desired mask pressure. These control methods need good software to accurately predict the system time delay, accurate sensor(s), and additional accessories to provide an effective control of the system.

None of these published patent control methods are suitable for a commercial product, as they neither consider patient comfort or production cost. In the following section a practical and commercially feasible method is discussed.

5.2 MATHEMATICAL MODELING

A lumped parameter model of the physical system and control elements is developed. A combination of analytical and empirical approaches is used.

5.2.1 Physical System

A typical CPAP system consists of a pressure-regulating valve, a thin tube, and a nasal mask. Figure 5-2 illustrates the connection, the manipulative desired input, and the measurable mask pressure output of such a system.

To simplify the modeling process, the pressure-regulating valve, thin tube, and the mask can be treated as one unit. The physical system is assumed to be a second order system, as higher order systems become too complex to be elegantly analyzed [7-9]. The physical system, as shown in Figure 5-3, may be represented by two time constants as in:

$$P_M = \frac{k_A}{(As+1)(Bs+1)} V_C \qquad (5-1)$$

where A and B are time constants of the physical system; k_A is the system gain; P_M is the mask pressure; s is the Laplace transform parameter; and V_C is the control voltage of the pressure-regulating valve.

Time delay is a common dynamic phenomenon associated with fluid flow. For tube lengths below 60 m the relationship between the lag and tube length is nearly linear [10]. The time delay between the two ends of the tube is equal to the fluid travel distance divided by the fluid velocity.

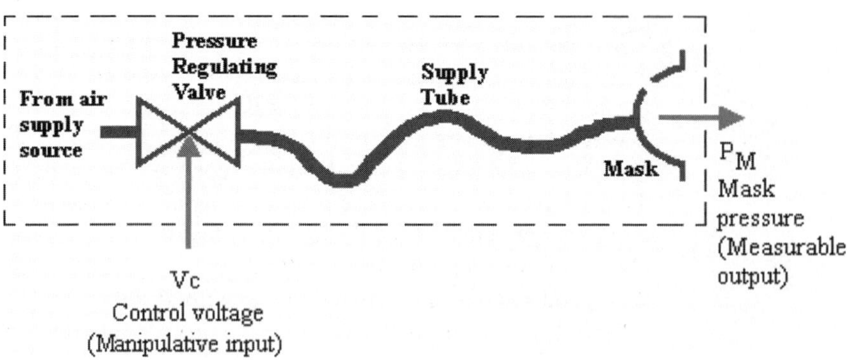

Figure 5-2. Schematic of a typical CPAP system

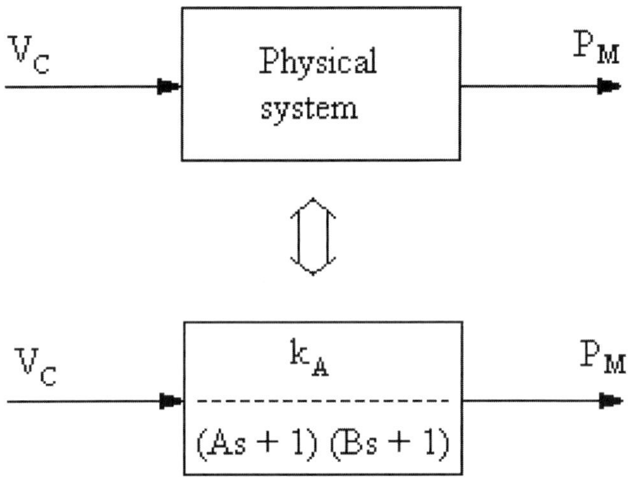

Figure 5-3. Process block and mathematical description of physical system

$$\text{Time Delay} = \frac{\text{Travel Distance}}{\text{Air Velocity}} \qquad (5-2)$$

It can be assumed that the density of the air inside the tube and the cross-sectional area of the tube are constant. For a standard breath cycle at rest combined with a typical bias flow of 50 L/min through the vent holes at the mask, the flow rate inside a 5.5-mm internal diameter supply air tube varies from 30 L/min to 90 L/min. Thus, the time delay in a 2-m-long supply tube will be approximately 30 ms to 90 ms, respectively. Time delay D_v also exists at the pressure-regulating valve, which must be added to the system in order to get the overall system delay.

Assuming that there is no time delay at the mask, the system time delay is not constant. It varies from $(30 + D_v)$ ms to $(90 + D_v)$ ms depending on the patients' breathing volume. An average time delay $(60 + D_v)$ ms will be used for the physical system for future simulation. Combining the time constant of the system and the average time delay, the overall physical system can be described by

$$P_M = V_C \frac{k_A}{(As+1)(Bs+1)} e^{-(0.06+D_v)s} \qquad (5-3)$$

5.2.2 Pressure Transducer

A pressure transducer is used to convert the measured pressure signal into a voltage signal. With careful selection, the response time of the pressure transducer can be very short (and hence neglected) and the output voltage of the pressure transducer is thus directly proportional to its measured pressure without any offset voltage. Such a pressure transducer can be modeled as a zero order device with no time delay. The output voltage of the pressure transducer is given by

$$V_T = k_T P_M \tag{5-4}$$

where V_T is the pressure transducer voltage output; k_T is the gain of the pressure transducer; and P_M is the mask pressure.

5.2.3 Controller

A proportional-integral-derivative (PID) type controller is used to control the physical system to maintain the constant mask pressure. The controller proportional gain, k_p, integral time, T_i, and derivative time, $T_{d,}$ can be adjusted to optimize the system performance. The ideal (standard) structure PID controller model is given by:

$$V_C = k_p\left(\mathrm{e} + \frac{1}{T_i}\int e dt + T_d \frac{de}{dt}\right) \tag{5-5}$$

Where V_C is the controller output and e is the error signal [11] to the controller. The error signal is equal to the difference between the desired and measured values of the controlled variable.

5.2.4 Breathing

The pressure variation due to breathing is considered as an independent input to the system. Measured data is used for this purpose.

5.3 SIMULINK™ MODEL

A Simulink™ model, which can be used to test and improve the control of the CPAP system, is given in this section.

5.3.1 Model Components

Figure 5-4 shows the block diagram of the overall system with feedback from the mask in terms of pressure. Figure 5-5 shows the overall system within Simulink™. The mask pressure is the controlled variable that is to be maintained within a specified range. The components or subsystems of the model are shown in Figure 5-6(a) to (d).

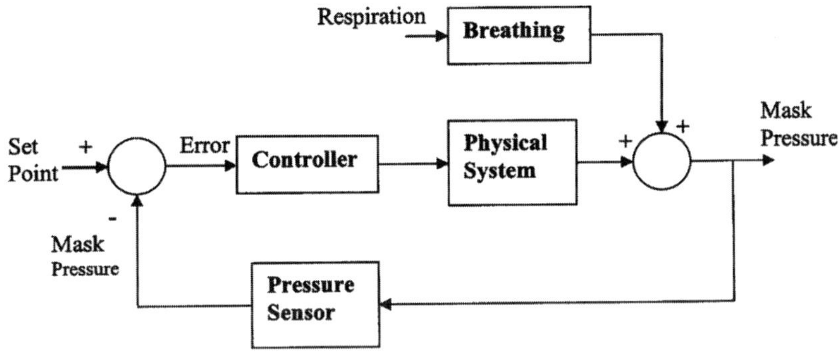

Figure 5-4. Block diagram of the overall system

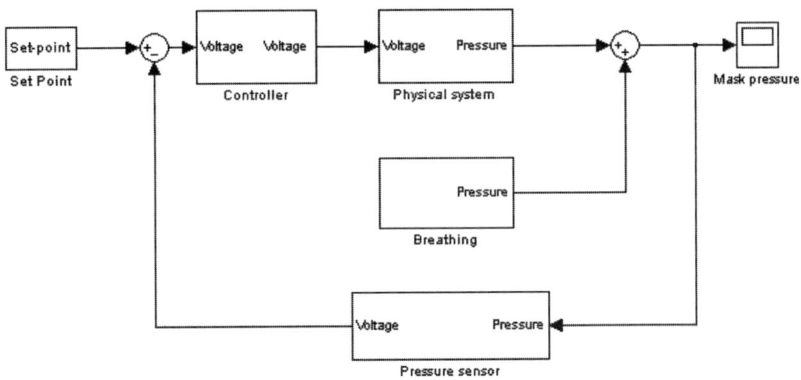

Figure 5-5. Overall system within Simulimk™

5.3.2 Open Loop Response

As a first step in the control analysis, the response of the original system to be controlled must be determined, in order to assess the possibility of achieving closed loop control. Table 5-1 gives the system constants that are used to simulate the basic model. These are derived from experimental results and typical equipment specifications [12].

TABLE 5-1. System constants

Constant	Description	Value	Units
A	Physical system time constant	0.025	second
B	Physical system time constant	0	second
k_A	Physical system gain	1.1	kPa/v
Dv	Time delay of pressure-regulating valve	0.007	second
k_T	Pressure transducer gain	1.6	v/kPa

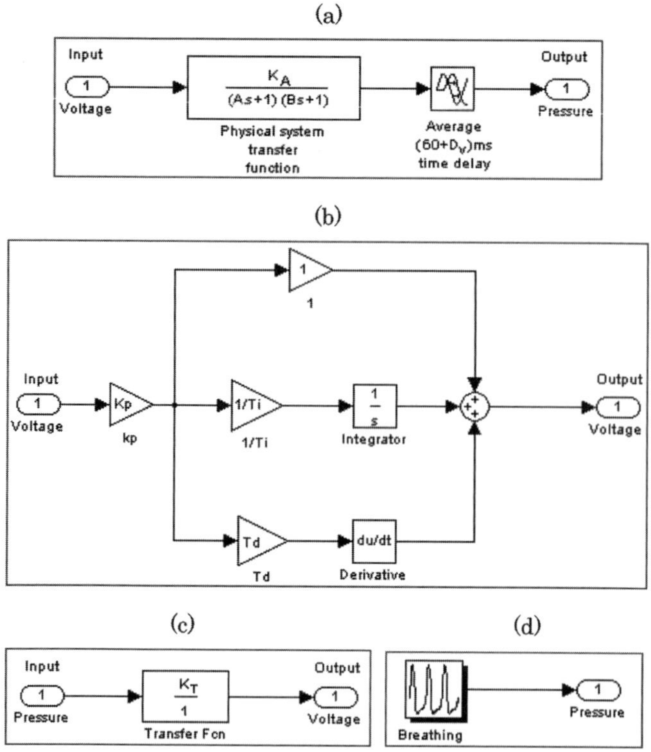

Figure 5-6. Model component: (a) physical system; (b) PID controller; (c) pressure transducer; and (d) breathing cycle

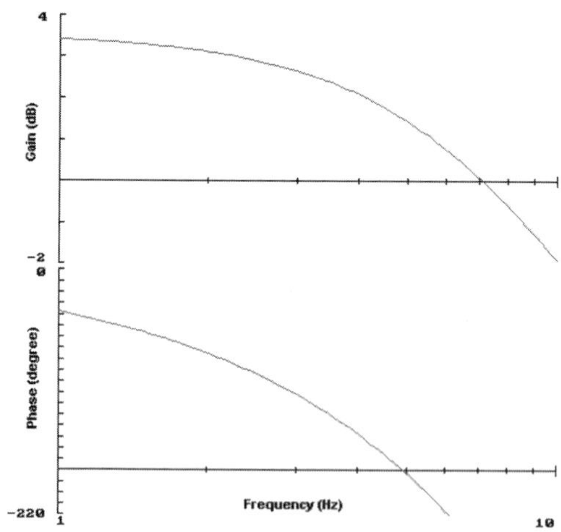

Figure 5-7. Bode plot of the overall system

The frequency response of the open loop system represented by the Bode plot is shown in Figure 5-7. This figure shows that the open loop gain is greater than unity at the frequency where the phase shift is greater than 180°. Thus this system is unstable for a closed loop system as the disturbance will grow in amplitude [13]. This instability is caused by the control system loop, and an improvement must be made to the basic system before it can be effectively controlled. Modeling techniques to achieve appropriate control parameters are discussed in the following sections.

5.4 APPROPRIATE CONTROL SCHEME

To achieve more accurate, dynamic, and adaptive control, a link or feedback path from the system output to the system input is required. A conventional feedback control as shown in Figure 5-8 may be considered. The main advantage of using negative feedback control is that it is unnecessary to know in advance what disturbances are likely to affect the mask pressure such as a cough, snore, or sneeze.

A pressure sensor installed at the mask transmits a voltage signal to the control system, which compares the received signal to the set point of the mask pressure. The algebraic difference between these two signals is the error signal. This error signal is then used as an input to the controller, which processes the signal to provide command action directly to the actuator. The controller output signal acts as an input to the process.

There are two methods to introduce system stability and control in a conventional feedback control loop with a time delay: (1) take the time

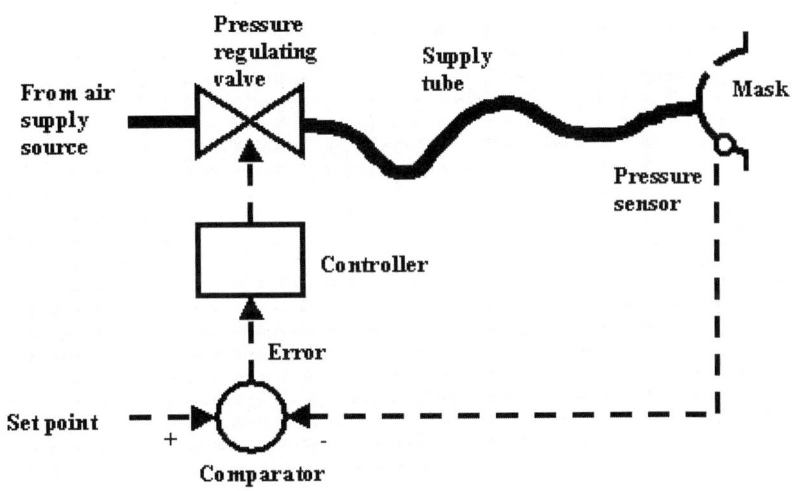

Figure 5-8. Schematic diagram of a possible control scheme

delay away from the feedback loop; or (2) eliminate the effect of the time delay in the feedback loop.

The first method, called "Time Constant Compensation," makes use of an electronic circuit connected in series to eliminate the effect of the time delay on the overall system. The second method, called "Time Delay Compensation," makes use of an electronic circuit connected in parallel to eliminate time delay from the feedback loop. These are presented in the following subsections as applied by Chan [12] to the present problem.

5.4.1 Time Constant Compensation

Figure 5-9 shows the block diagram connection of the Time Constant Compensation Circuit (TCCC). The open loop gain and time constant of the physical system can be determined by experimental measurements where the response of the pressure sensor at the mask is determined as a result of a step input to the pressure regulating valve. Typical values for such a device are an open loop gain of 1.1 and a time constant of 25 ms [12].

The TCCC is placed between the controller and the physical system. It is a first order transfer function with a long time constant, Tc, which is 10 times longer than the time constant of the physical system. The TCCC combines with the physical system to become a second order system with an average 67 ms system time delay. The pole of the TCCC can be considered as the dominant pole [7] of the combined system, as it is at least 10 times closer to the origin than the pole of the physical system.

It is common practice that if the real part of a pole is at least 5 to 10 times that of a dominant pole or a pair of complex dominant poles, then

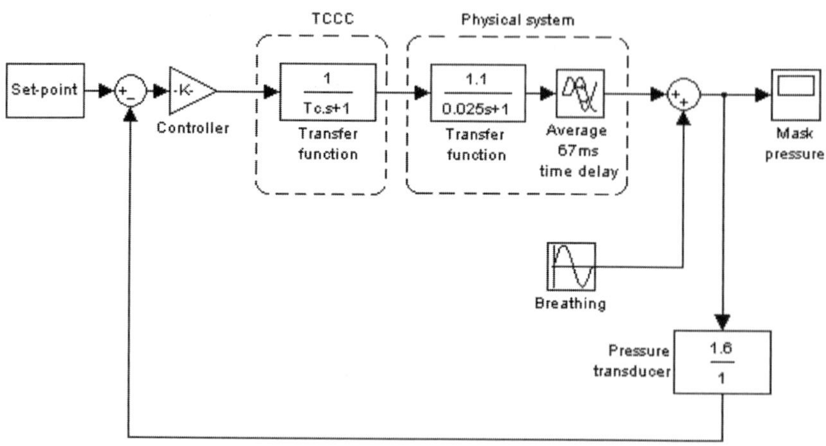

Figure 5-9. TCCC connection block diagram

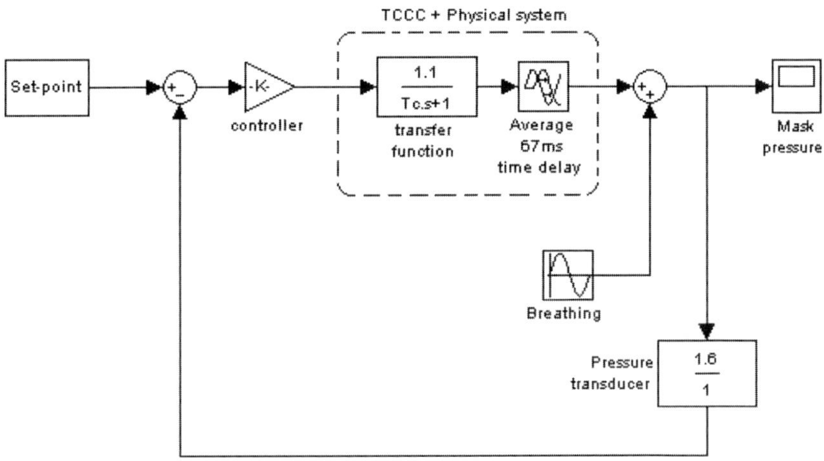

Figure 5-10. Simplified block diagram with TCCC

the pole may be regarded as insignificant insofar as the transient is concerned [13]. Therefore, the pole of the physical system can be considered as having very little or no effect on the system. Thus, the pole of the actual system can be neglected, and the overall system can be simplified to a first order system with a time delay. A resultant simplified block diagram is shown in Figure 5-10.

Figure 5-11 shows the simulation of the closed loop system with time delay compensation. The model simulation reveals that for a 0.5 kPa mask

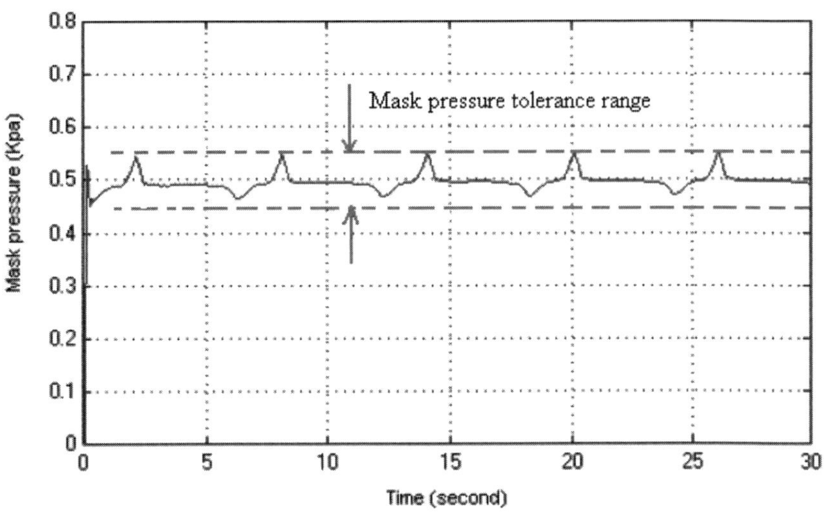

Figure 5-11. Computer simulation result of TCCC

pressure set point, the maximum mask pressure fluctuation remains within the typically desired limits of 0.05 kPa. The settings required to meet the said optimum response are k_p=15, T_i=0.1 s, T_d=0.025 s, and T_c=1.5 s.

5.4.2 Time Delay Compensation

The Time Delay Compensation Circuit (TDCC) is designed to remove time delay from the feedback loop. Figure 5-12 shows how a parallel circuit consisting of two transfer functions and a gain controller is equivalent to the physical system itself. The time constant and gain values of the model transfer functions are redistributed in order to match the combined values of the physical system. The controller output forms inputs to both the model transfer function and to the physical system. The output signal from the model transfer function and time delay cancels the feedback signal from the pressure transducer. If the model is perfect, the output signal of summer 1 will be zero, and no error signal is fed back to the controller.

The output signal from the model transfer function before the model time delay is a model signal without time delay and can thus be used to predict the output of the actual mask pressure. This output signal can be used as feedback to the controller to fine-tune the mask pressure as shown in Figure 5-13.

Perfect matching is unrealistic even in computer simulations. In practice, the output from summer 1 is the modeling error between the

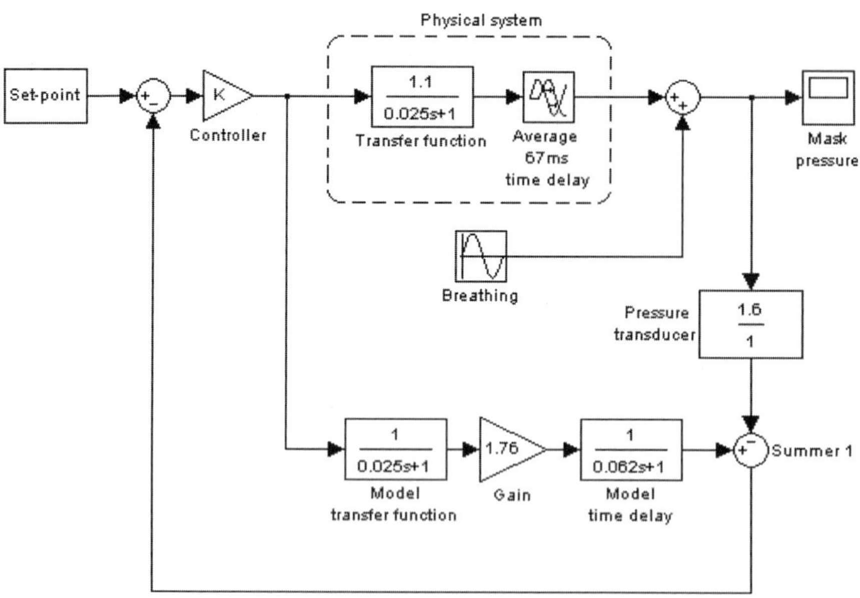

Figure 5-12. Feedback loop cancellation

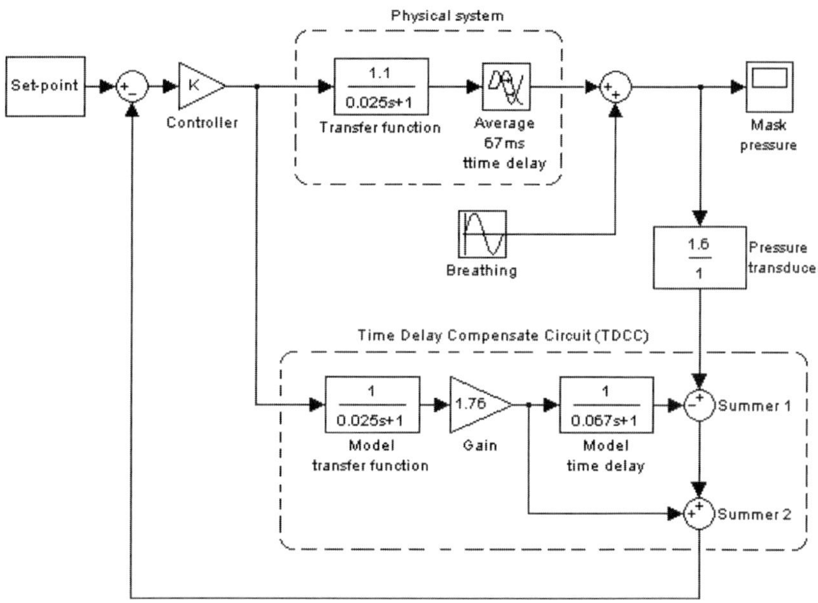

Figure 5-13. Time delay compensation

actual system and the model transfer functions. This error signal will be added to the feedback path and input to the controller.

The general overall operation, with perfect modeling, is shown with the aid of the equivalent circuit in Figure 5-14. The system time delay is outside the feedback loop, which consists of the transfer function of physical system and the controller. The system can therefore be tuned tightly.

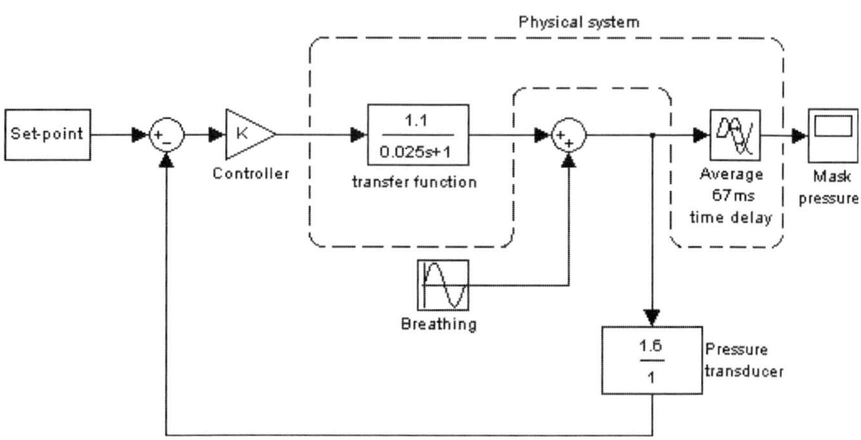

Figure 5-14. Equivalent loop for perfect matching

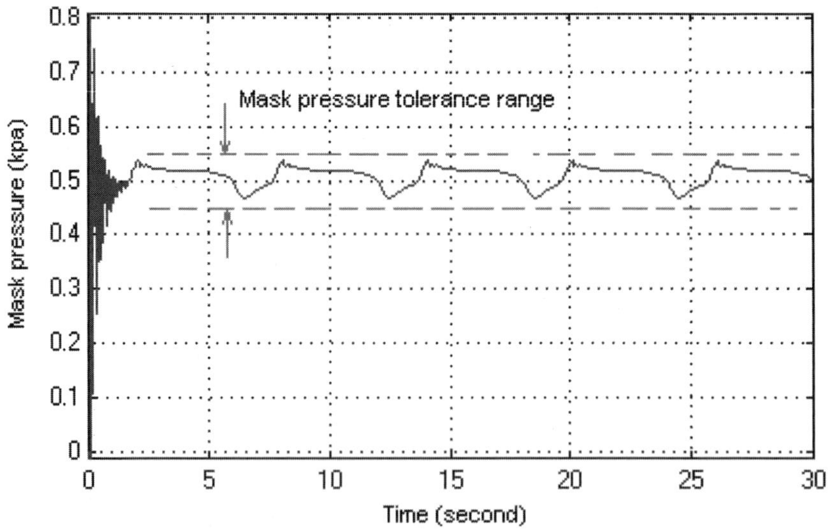

Figure 5-15. Computer simulation result of TDCC

The optimum fluctuations in mask pressure as determined from model simulations are shown in Figure 5-15. Initially, there is a 60% overshoot in mask pressure. The system takes approximately 2 seconds to reach steady state, where the variation remains within the desired limits of +/- 0.05 kPa for a 0.5-kPa mask pressure set point after steady state is reached. The settings required to meet the optimum response are k_p= 7, T_i=0.1 s, and T_d=0.025 s.

A widely accepted control paradigm in practice is to adjust the controller so that the response of the system has an amplitude ratio or decay ratio of one-quarter. A decay ratio of one-quarter means that the ratio of two successive overshoots is four to one.

5.5 CONTROLLER TUNING

Techniques for adjusting controllers are classified as either open-loop or closed-loop methods. A good control paradigm is to adjust the controller so that the response of the system has an amplitude ratio or decay ratio of one-quarter. Ziegler and Nichols [14] proposed a decay ratio of one-quarter, which means that the ratio of two successive overshoots is four to one.

Techniques for adjusting controllers are classified as either open loop or closed loop methods. The tuning procedure that uses the result from an open-loop test is called the "reaction curve method." The second method derived from the same source is called the "continuous cycling method," which uses a closed loop test.

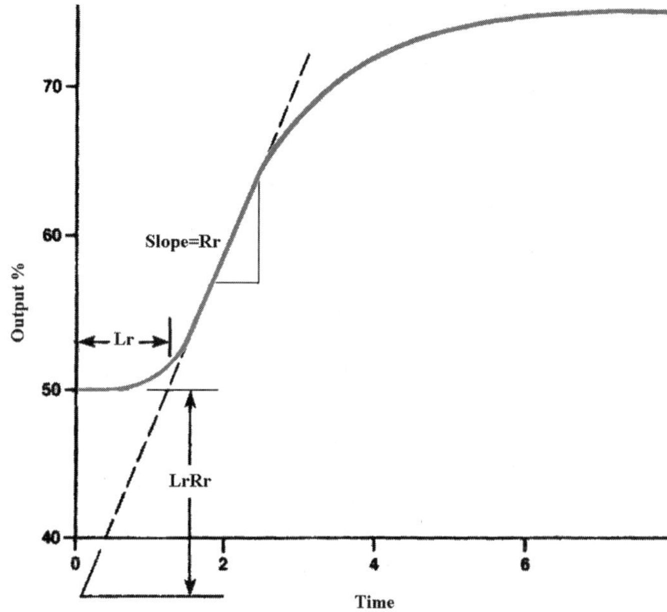

Figure 5-16. Reaction curve

5.5.1 Reaction Curve Method

The reaction curve is the response of the process to a step change in its input. To use the reaction curve method, the first step is to determine the process reaction rate, Rr, and the process lag, Lr, from the reaction curve.

A tangent is drawn to the process reaction curve at its point of maximum slope as illustrated in Figure 5-16. This slope is the process reaction rate, Rr. The intersection of this tangent with the original base line gives an indication of the process lag, Lr, which is an equivalent time delay of the process. If this tangent drawn at the point of maximum slope is extrapolated to a vertical axis drawn at the time when the step is imposed, then the amount by which this is below the horizontal base line will represent the product LrRr.

By knowing these parameters the controller can be tuned by referring to the controller settings given in Table 5-2. Due to the difficulty faced in determining the point of maximum slope, and the equivalent time delay, and the complication faced due to noise in practical measurements, this method is not very effective.

5.5.2 Continuous Cycling Method

The continuous cycling method is also called the "ultimate cycle method." The term "ultimate" is used to determine the ultimate gain and ultimate period for the loop. For a feedback control system, if the loop is closed

TABLE 5-2. Controller parameters

	Reaction Curve Method			Continuous Cycling Method		
	k_p	T_i	T_d	k_p	T_i	T_d
Proportional only	l/LrRr	-	-	0.5 Su	-	-
Proportional-plus-integral	0.9/LrRr	3.33 Lr	-	0.45 Su	Pu/l.2	-
Proportional-plus-integral-plus-derivative	1.2/LrRr	2.0 Lr	0.5 Lr	0.6 Su	0.5 Pu	Pu/8

and the controller is on automatic mode, increasing the controller gain will cause the loop to oscillate. If the controller gain increases further, the system will oscillate continuously. The maximum gain at which the system is operated before it becomes unstable is the ultimate gain. The period of these sustained oscillations is the ultimate period. If the controller gain is increased further, the system will become unstable. These general situations are as shown in Figure 5-17.

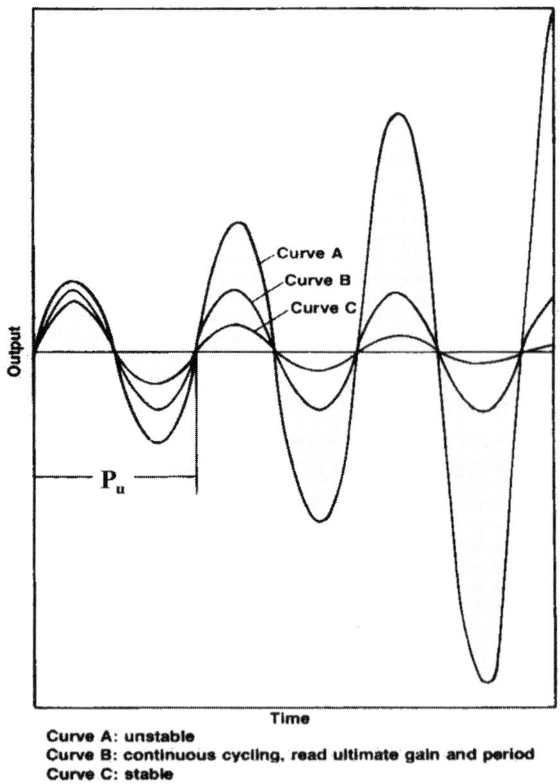

Figure 5-17. Response to illustrate ultimate gain and ultimate period

The following steps are used to determine the ultimate gain and the ultimate period:

1. Disable all the integral and derivative action from the controller, leaving only the proportional mode. This may be achieved by setting T_i equal to infinity and T_d equal to zero, or as close to these values as possible.
2. Maintain the controller on automatic mode and leave the loop closed.
3. With the gain of the proportional mode of the controller at some arbitrary value, impose a disturbance on the process and observe the response. A method for imposing this disturbance is to move the set point for a few seconds and then return it to its original value.
4. If the response curve from Step 3 does not damp out (as in Curve A in Figure 5-17), the gain is too high; the gain should be decreased and Step 3 repeated.
5. If the response curve in Step 3 damps out (as in Curve C in Figure 5-17), the gain is too low; the gain should be increased and Step 3 repeated.
6. When a response curve similar to Curve B in Figure 5-17 is obtained, the values of the ultimate gain setting and the ultimate period of the associated response curve are noted. This ultimate gain at which the sustained oscillations are encountered is the ultimate sensitivity, Su, and the ultimate period is Pu.
7. The ultimate gain and the ultimate period are then used to calculate controller settings. By knowing these parameters the controller can be tuned by referring to the controller settings in Table 5-2.

5.6 FLOW SENSORS

Sensors are used at several positions within the CPAP system for various applications. While some are used for control purposes, such as the pressure sensor in Section 5.2, others are used for monitoring purposes to achieve optimum comfort for the patient. Appendix B gives a summary of various sensing devices and their suitability for use in the CPAP system. As an example of sensor selection, this section summarizes a procedure to select a hotwire anemometer as a flow sensor, which could be used to determine whether the patient is actually using the device and to measure dynamic signals of the patient's breath cycle for breath disorder diagnostics. The section intends to help improve understanding of airflow measurement within a CPAP device and investigate the characteristics of a selected airflow sensor.

Assume that it is desired to determine the characteristics for a hotwire anemometer to measure the air flow velocity for the purpose of breath cycle diagnostics. The sensor is considered to be a first order device that can be represented by [15]:

$$\frac{e}{V} = \frac{K}{\tau D + 1} \quad (5-6)$$

where e and V are output voltage and input velocity, respectively. The static sensitivity K and time constant τ can be defined by:

$$K = \frac{A_w K_v (K_{tr} R_{w0} - T_a)}{i_w^2 - A_w K_{tr} h} \quad (5-7)$$

and

$$\tau = \frac{M C_w K_{tr}}{A_w K_{tr} h - i_w^2} \quad (5-8)$$

where i_w is the current flow through the wire; $R_{w0,}$ r_w, A_w, M, and C_w, are the initial resistance, change in resistance, surface area, mass and specific heat of the hot wire, respectively; K_v is the coefficient of flow velocity (variation of h with respect to velocity determined at a reference velocity); K_{tr} is the reciprocal of a temperature coefficient of wire resistance; T_a is the air temperature; and h is the convective heat transfer coefficient.

Before proceeding with the selection criterion, some accuracy conditions are imposed on the sensor. Assume this sensor is designed to measure a patient's breath cycle for diagnosing the severity of obstructive sleep apnea (OSA). The experimental breath cycle used in Chapters 2 and 3 can take different forms for various OSA conditions. With a breathing rate of 14 breaths per minute and looking at the first 14 harmonics of the breath cycle, a frequency of 3.27 (14x14/60) Hz should be considered. Using this frequency and 3 dB signal accuracy limit, the amplitude ratio would be 0.708. Using this value in equation (5-6) gives:

$$\frac{1}{\sqrt{\omega^2 \tau^2 + 1}} = \frac{1}{\sqrt{(2\pi \times 3.27)^2 \tau^2 + 1}} \geq 0.708 \quad (5-9)$$

The last equation gives a maximum value of the time constant τ to be 49 ms, which is the duration required to differentiate between a normal and an abnormal breath cycle.

To determine the actual time constant, however, the following procedure may be followed:

1. To determine the convective heat transfer characteristics of the sensor, determination of whether the flow is laminar or turbulent is necessary. To avoid fluid obstructions and reduce loading effects, a very thin wire must be selected. The minimum commercially available platinum wire diameter, d, is 0.02 mm. From previous chapters, the range of air velocity V_{air} in a CPAP

machine is less than 10 m/s. Knowing the kinematic viscosity of air at room temperature of 1.55x10^{-5} results in a very small Reynolds number, $R_e = Vd/v$, indicating that the flow can be assumed laminar.

2. To determine the forced convection heat transfer coefficient, h, it is necessary to determine the Nusselt number N_u and the Prandtl number P_r. Assuming the wire as a cylinder in cross flow, the formulas for these numbers are given by [16]:

$$N_u = \frac{hd}{k} = 0.3 + \frac{0.62 R_e^{1/2} \cdot P_r^{1/3}}{[1 + (0.40 / P_r)^{2/3}]^{1/4}} \left[1 + \left(\frac{R_e}{282{,}000} \right)^{5/8} \right]^{4/5} \qquad (5-10)$$

where k is the thermal conductivity and

$$P_r = \frac{v}{\alpha} = \frac{\mu C_p}{k} \qquad (5-11)$$

where α is the thermal diffusivity; μ is the air viscosity; and C_p is the specific heat capacity of air at constant pressure. Combining equation (5-10) with equation (5-11) leads to the following equation of forced convective coefficient h [16, 17]:

$$h = \frac{k \times 0.989 \times \left(\frac{V_{air} \times \sin\theta \times d}{v} \right)^{0.330} \times \left(\frac{\mu C_p}{k} \right)^{1/3}}{d} \qquad (5-12)$$

where V_{air} is the air velocity, which is inclined at an angle of θ from the wire.

3. To determine the other constants in equation (5-8), the resistance R_w for a platinum wire can be written as [16]:

$$R_w = R_0(1 + a \times (T_w - 273) + b \times (T_w - 273)^2) \qquad (5-13)$$

Where R_0 is the wire resistance at 0°C, T_w is the wire temperature, and the value of coefficient b is 3.9083×10^{-3} and that of a is $^-5.665 \times 10^{-7}$. The wire resistance R_w in terms of the wire resistivity Kr_t can be expressed as:

$$R_w = Kr_t \times L / A \qquad (5-14)$$

Using this equation and equation (5-13), the resistivity Kr_t can be determined from:

$$Kr_t = \frac{R_0(1 + a \times (T_w - 273) + b \times (T_w - 273)^2) \times A}{L} \qquad (5-15)$$

Using the above constants and ignoring small terms, this equation may reduce to:

$$Kr_t = 0.0365 \times 10^{-8} \times T_w \qquad (5-16)$$

Substituting this equation into equation (5-14) results in:

$$R_w = 0.0365 \times 10^{-8} \times T_w \times L/(\pi \cdot r^2) \qquad (5-17)$$

where L and r are the length and radius of the wire, respectively. Rearranging this equation to get the reciprocal of the temperature coefficient K_{tr} as

$$K_{tr} = \frac{T_w}{R_w} = \frac{(\pi \cdot r^2)}{3.65 \times 10^{-10} \times L} \qquad (5-18)$$

This equation can be used to simulate a general model for the hot wire. However, if equation (5-12) is differentiated with respect to the air velocity and using the platinum wire characteristics, the result is:

$$K_v = 413.33 \times V^{-0.6697} \qquad (5-19)$$

4. Assume that the small platinum wire of 0.02 mm diameter is suitably fitted in a typical air delivery tube of 20 mm diameter (ratio of 1/100). Using a flow rate of 0.0314 L/s within the tube gives an air velocity of 1 m/s. Substituting this value into equation (5-8) gives a time constant of 22 ms. This time constant value is much smaller than the maximum value of 49 ms, which was previously determined. However, for practical purposes, the sensor strength and its capability to sustain forces due to airflow must be considered before the sensor is actually fitted in the system. This is a standard design step; however, it is beyond the scope of this book.

5.7 CLOSURE

This chapter deals with the modeling of a typical CPAP system for the purposes of developing a control scheme for regulating pressure in the mask. A brief introduction of available control schemes is given. The CPAP system and controller are then modeled in Simulink™ to determine an appropriate controller scheme and settings. Techniques for tuning the controller are also discussed.

REFERENCES

[1] Sleep Apnoea Breathing Therapy - Part 1: Sleep Apnoea Breathing Therapy Devices (Adopted ISO 17510-1:2002, first edition, 2002–02-01). 2002: Canadian Standards Association.

[2] Sorkin, I.B., Rapoport, D. M., Method And Apparatus For The Treatment Of Obstructive Sleep Apnea, U.S.o.A.P. Office, Editor. 1987.

[3] Lynch, C., Sullivan, C. D., Method And Apparatus Useful In The Diagnosis Of Obstructive Sleep Apnea Of A Patient, U.S.o.A.P. Office, Editor. 2002.

[4] Stenzler, A., Infant CPAP System With Airway Pressure Control, U.S.o.A.P. Office, Editor. 2002.

[5] Berthon, J.M., Lynch, E. C., CPAP Respiratory Apparatus, U.S.o.A.P. Office, Editor. 2002.

[6] Berthon, J.M., Detection Of Apnea, E.P. Office, Editor. 1999.

[7] Golten, J., Verwer, A., Control System Design and Simulation International Edition. 1992, Singapore: McGraw-Hill Book Co.

[8] Davison, E.J., A Method for Simplifying Linear Dynamic System. IEEE Trans Automatic Contro, 1966. **AC-11**: p. 93–101.

[9] Hsia, T.C., The Simplification of Linear System. IEEE Trans. Automatic Control, 1972. **AC-17**: p. 372–374.

[10] Shinskey, F.G., Process-Control Systems Application/Design/Adjustment. 2nd ed. 1979, New York: McGraw Hill Book Company.

[11] Johnson, C.D., Process Control Instrumentation Technology. 5th ed. 1997, New York: Prentice-Hall International Inc.

[12] Chan, H.K., Control Scheme for Sleep Apnea Treatment Devices, Master of Engineering thesis, 2004. Auckland University of Technology.

[13] Kuo, B.C., Automatic Control Systems. 6th ed. 1991: Prentice-Hall International Editions.

[14] Ziegler, J.G., Nichols, N.B., Optimum Settings for Automatic Controllers. Trans ASME, 1942. **64**: p. 759–68.

[15] Doebelin, E.O., Measurement Systems: Application and Design. 5th ed. 2004: McGraw Hill.

[16] Bejan, A., Kraus, A.D., Heat Transfer Handbook. 2003: John Wiley & Sons.

[17] Thomas, L.C., Heat Transfer-Professional Version. 1999: Capstone Publishing Corporation.

Chapter 6

MASK DESIGN

This chapter covers typical fluid, thermodynamic, and computational fluid dynamic models that are used to determine condensation in masks used in Continuous Positive Airway Pressure (CPAP) devices. First, the fundamental mechanisms of condensation and carbon dioxide (CO_2) generation in CPAP masks are addressed, as well as possible design solutions to effectively control these in practice. The utility of mathematical and computational models is then demonstrated by using them to determine design parameters and condensation levels and locations in a typical mask.

6.1 BASIC PRINCIPLES OF CONDENSATION AND CARBON DIOXIDE

Air breathers deliver air under pressure into the nostrils, and the airflow acts as a pneumatic splint that keeps the pharyngeal airway open so that the humidified fresh air can get through the airway into the lung. The mask is the main interface between the patient and the breathing system and is considered the key component that affects the patient's comfort. Problems such as high carbon dioxide concentration and condensation discourage and limit mask use. Industrial research has been undertaken in order to address these issues. Previous work suggests [1] that reducing the steady state background pressure of CO_2 can alleviate central apnea. Thus, optimizing mask design and taking into consideration the patient's comfort is an important step in the acceptance of the CPAP system.

Some research suggests that custom-fabricated masks [2] aimed at minimizing skin pressure and discomfort can be used to fit an individual patient. However, limitations that include a complicated production process, high cost, and durability make mass production impossible.

The deposition of the bias flow ports also affects the CO_2 ventilation. Studies by Schettino [3] revealed that placing the exhalation port within the mask and minimizing volume results in less CO_2 re-breathing simply due to the shorter route for CO_2 residing in the mask.

In general, there are several types of air delivery masks available on the market, each with certain features preferred by the users. However, these masks may be categorized under four types of delivery (see Figure 6-1):

1. Nasal delivery
2. Full face delivery
3. Direct Nasal delivery
4. Oral delivery

The advantages and disadvantages of these masks are identified by manufacturer's catalogs and are beyond the scope of this book. In general, user comfort decides what type of mask to use. Nevertheless, some of these types have encountered problems in use. For example, a full face mask is normally preferred over a nasal mask as it is believed that the latter may cause a leaky mouth during sleep, which may result in a dry nose and throat. On the other hand, face masks can result in marks and pressure on the user's face, which could be the main elements of discomfort.

A typical breather mask contains arrays of orifices to expel the exhaled air to ensure that the patient can breathe the fresh air delivered by the humidifier. The diameters of the orifices are generally determined by the bias flow rate required at minimum pressure to clear the CO_2 inside the mask. It is believed that higher gas flow rates are necessary to retain a relatively low inspiratory CO_2 concentration [4]. However, experimental measurements [5] show that the inspiratory fraction of CO_2 is minimized below 0.5% as long as the bias flow rate is maintained above 15 L/min. For a fixed bias flow orifice diffuser system, the bias flow rate increases as the breather's pressure increases. This suggests that the bias flow rate at a high pressure setting is much higher than that required in terms of CO_2 ventilation. The higher bias flow rate normally produces noise and an increased pressure swing. The higher noise disturbs the patient's sleep and increases pressure swings, which elevates the patient's breathing load.

A fixed bias flow rate adequate enough to maintain low CO_2 concentration for the entire pressure range may solve these issues. Adjusting the bias flow characteristics may not only affect the circulation of CO_2, but also facilitate the expulsion of vapor exhaled from patients. As a result, this will help reduce condensation inside the mask.

During normal operation conditions, the breather humidifier continuously supplies moisturized air to the patient. The relative humidity inside the mask is maintained at a modest level so that patients do not develop dry throats when wearing the mask over a period of hours. In general, the more stagnant vapor there is inside the mask, the more condensation is likely to occur. Condensation also occurs frequently during the night when the room temperature is relatively low.

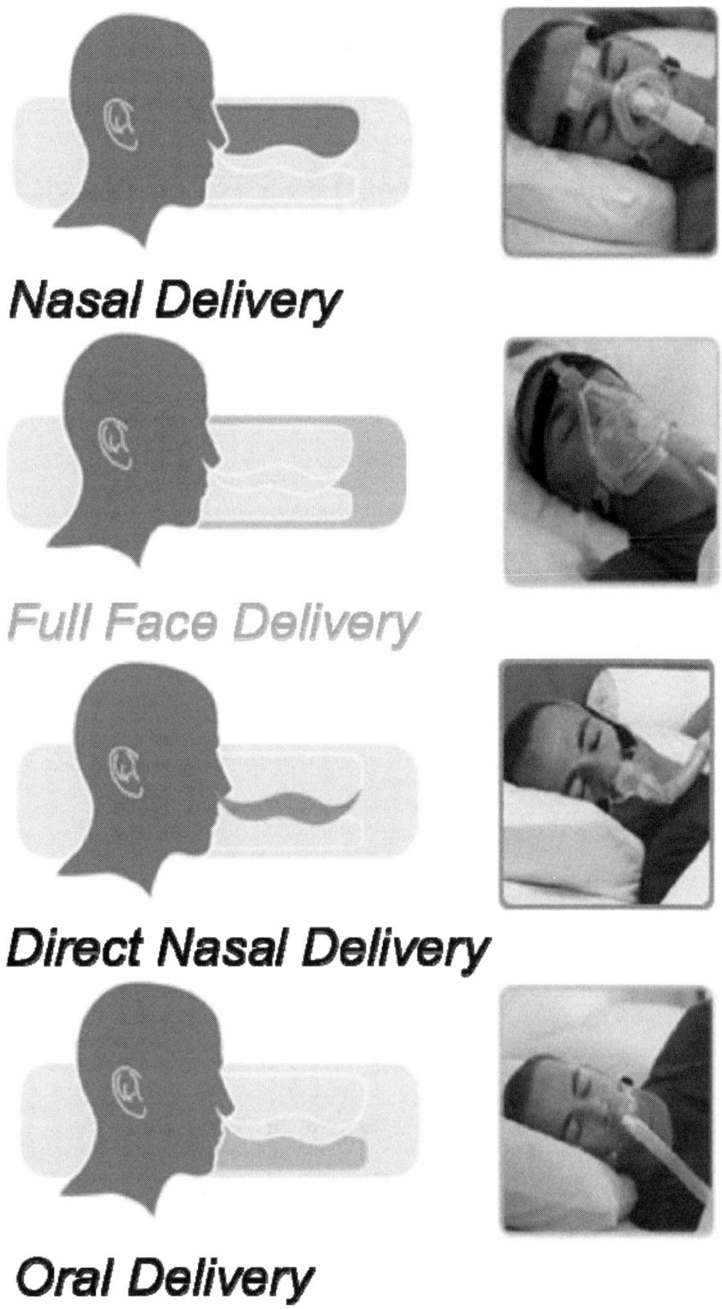

Figure 6-1. Typical masks [Courtesy of Fisher & Paykel Healthcare Ltd]

One way to reduce condensation is to keep the relative humidity low, or raise the inside surface temperature above the saturation temperature. However, adjusting the position of the bias flow orifice in order to provide better ventilation is believed to be as effective as the aforementioned two methods.

6.2 MATHEMATICAL MODELS TO DETERMINE DESIGN PARAMETERS

Every breather mask has a ventilation mechanism to maintain fresh air within. This is called the orifice diffuser or bias flow system. The primary function of the orifice diffuser system is to maintain air circulation by expelling exhaled air to the surrounding ambient, while fresh air is supplied to the mask to ensure that there is no re-breathing. This helps to maintain a low CO_2 concentration inside the mask.

To design the mask geometry, in this section a typical fluid dynamic model of an orifice diffuser system is presented to correlate pressure with the effective orifice area and the bias flow rate.

6.2.1 Fluid Modeling

The orifice flow rate, Q, is derived from the well-known Bernoulli's equation and is proportional to the orifice cross-sectional area, A, and the square root of the pressure drop, P (see Figure 6-2).

$$Q = C_d A \sqrt{\frac{2}{\rho} P} \tag{6-1}$$

where the discharge coefficient, C_d, is determined by:

$$Cd = \frac{C_v C_c}{\sqrt{1 - Cc^2 (A_{vc}/A_u)^2}} \tag{6-2}$$

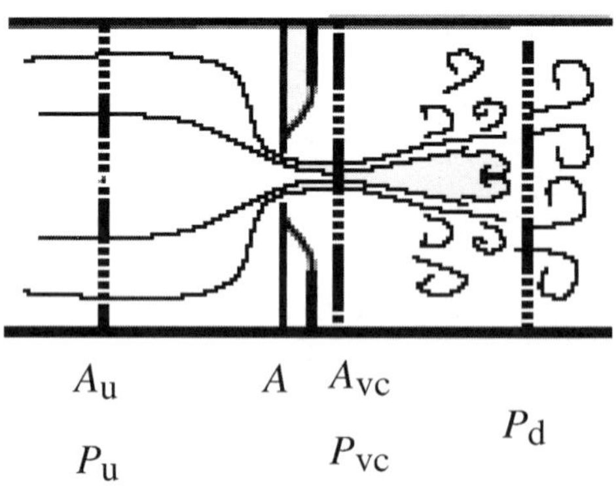

Figure 6-2. Flow through an orifice

where C_v is the flow velocity coefficient; C_c is area contraction coefficient; A_{vc} is the cross-sectional area at the vena contracta; A_u is the cross-sectional area located upstream; and P is the pressure differential between the pressure upstream, P_u, and the pressure at vena contracta, P_{vc}.

If $A_u \gg A$, then $(A/A_u)^2 \rightarrow 0$ and the discharge coefficient $C_d = C_v C_c$. The discharge coefficient, C_d, is often assumed to be constant and independent of the Reynolds number. However, a mask's bias flow represents an orifice diffuser system with very small holes to reduce noisy draft inside the mask. For such orifices the discharge coefficient is not constant anymore and needs to be determined.

The Reynolds number for a bias flow diffuser system is defined as:

$$\mathrm{Re} = \frac{\rho(Q/A)D_h}{\mu} \tag{6-3}$$

where D_h is the tube diameter; ρ is the fluid density; and μ is the fluid absolute viscosity.

Wu [6] suggests the following empirical model for a variety of orifices with different geometries covering laminar to turbulent flow regimes:

$$Cd = Cd_\infty \left(1 + ae^{-\frac{\delta 1}{Cd_\infty}\sqrt{\mathrm{Re}}} + be^{-\frac{\delta 2}{Cd_\infty}\sqrt{\mathrm{Re}}}\right) \tag{6-4}$$

where Cd_∞ is the turbulent discharge coefficient for a specific orifice; $\delta 1$ and $\delta 2$ are the laminar discharge coefficients; and a and b are shape dependent coefficients to be determined.

For the breather diffuser system, the following conditions are assumed to determine the four constants $\delta 1$, $\delta 2$, a, and b.

1. Initially when there is no flow, C_d should be set to zero. This gives:

$$C_d\big|_{\sqrt{\mathrm{Re}}=0} = 1 + a + b = 0 \tag{6-5}$$

2. The laminar discharge coefficient can be obtained by assuming $\frac{\partial C_d}{\partial\sqrt{\mathrm{Re}}}$ equals a constant δ such that:

$$\frac{\partial C_d}{\partial\sqrt{\mathrm{Re}}}\bigg|_{\sqrt{\mathrm{Re}=0}} = -a\delta 1 - b\delta 2 = \delta \tag{6-6}$$

3. Assuming *Rem* represents the Reynolds number where the discharge coefficient is at a maximum, i.e.

$$Cdm = Cd\infty\left(1 + ae^{-\frac{\delta 1}{Cd_\infty}\sqrt{Rem}} + 1 + be^{-\frac{\delta 2}{Cd_\infty}\sqrt{Rem}}\right) \tag{6-7}$$

The maximum C_d is determined by setting the differentiation of C_d with respect to *Re* to zero:

$$\frac{\partial Cd}{\partial\sqrt{\text{Re}}}\bigg|_{\sqrt{\text{Re}}=0} = -a\delta 1 e^{-\frac{\delta 1}{Cd_\infty}\sqrt{Rem}} - b\delta 2 e^{-\frac{\delta 2}{Cd_\infty}\sqrt{Rem}} = 0 \qquad (6-8)$$

4. Equations (6-5) to (6-8) can be solved simultaneously to determine δ1, δ2, *a*, and *b*; however, $C_{d\infty}$, C_{dm}, Rem, and δ need to be determined experimentally. Typical values are $C_{d\infty}=0.61$, $C_{dm}=0.69$, Rem $=121$, and $\delta = 0.23$ [6]. Using these values gives a typical discharge coefficient of the form:

$$C_d = 0.61(1+1.07e^{-0.126\sqrt{\text{Re}}} - 2.07e^{-0.246\sqrt{\text{Re}}}) \qquad (6-9)$$

The formula compares well with experimental values by Merritt [7], which are widely accepted in industrial research. See Figure 6-3.

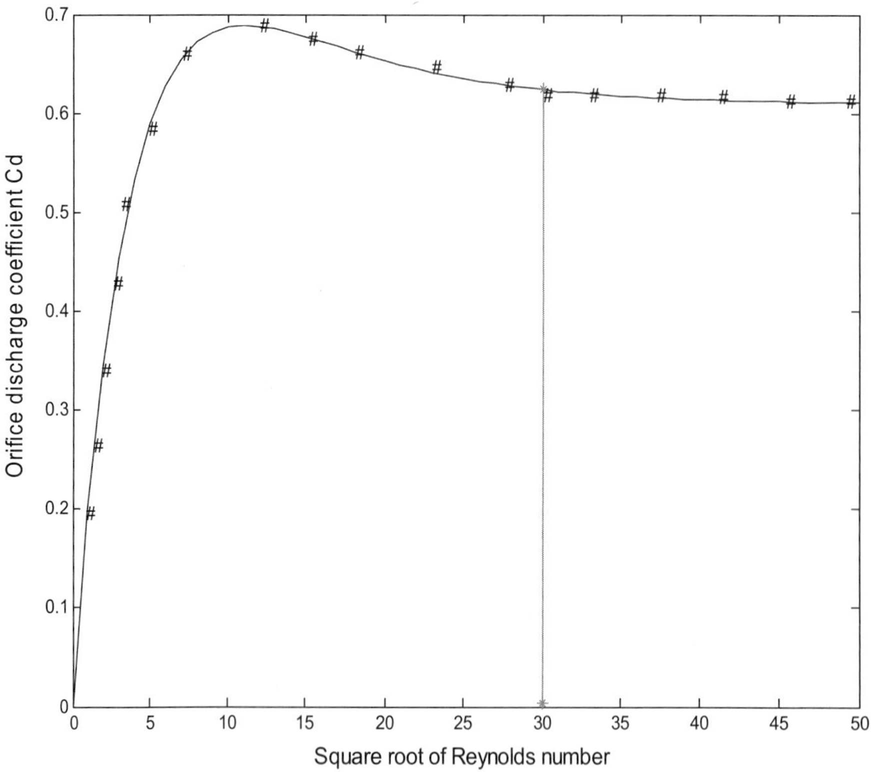

Figure 6-3. Comparison between empirical orifice model and experimental data from Merritt [7]

The model shows that there is no appreciable degree of variation for C_d if the Reynolds number is maintained between 900 and 2500. The discharge coefficient may be considered as constant in that range. This suggests that a careful design is required to ensure that parameters such as D_h and A are selected in such a way that the Reynolds number remains within this range.

6.2.2 Design Considerations of Pressure and Area Effects

In most fluid systems, flow control is mainly accomplished by throttling flow through the orifice. As indicated by the flow rate equation (6-1), effectively adjusting the area of the diffuser system in response to the pressure change is the most viable way to produce a constant bias flow rate.

A constant bias flow rate can be achieved by using a feedback control in the breather itself. This would normally introduce a complicated control scheme including a battery and sensors, and so it involves extra manufacturing costs. A more viable way to regulate the bias flow rate is by mechanically adjusting the effective area of the orifice diffuser system. Based on the flow rate equation (6-1), an orifice with an adjustable area inversely proportional to the square root of the pressure would be ideal. However, such mechanisms that produce satisfactory outcomes have not been found in the literature.

Alternatively, novel designs that approximate this behavior may be used to accomplish a constant bias flow. An example is that of Zhen [5], where an adjustable orifice area is achieved by changing the gap between the diaphragm and valve as seen in Figure 6-4. The deformation of the diaphragm is enabled by cutting four small slots into it.

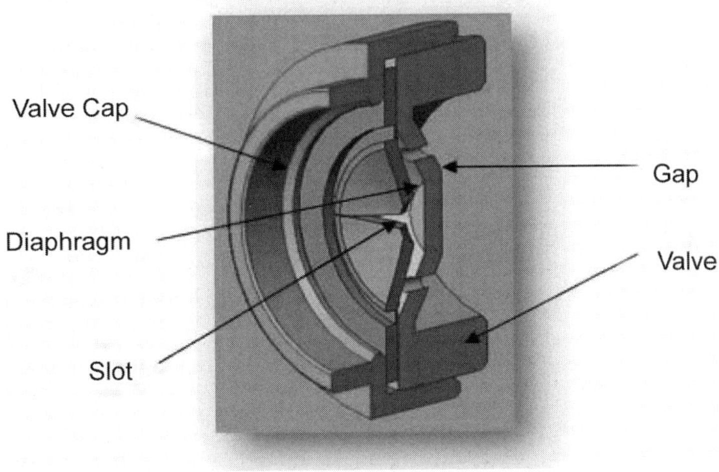

Figure 6-4. Isometric section of orifice diffuser design [5]

6.3 MODELING CONDENSATION

Humidified air in the mask offers comfortable breathing conditions to patients with obstructive sleep apnea, while avoiding a dry throat. When the vapor temperature on the inside surface of the mask is lower than its saturation temperature, condensation occurs. This condensation disturbs the patient's sleep, and compromises the patient's acceptance of CPAP treatment.

Excessive condensation on the mask surface normally indicates that the humidity level inside the mask is too high. The relative humidity is a function of moisture in the air and the temperature. The higher the relative humidity of the air near the mask, the higher the dew point temperature will be at that particular area. As a result, warm air holds more moisture.

Condensation phenomenon has been an area of research for over a hundred years, and it is believed that the best way to control condensation is to keep the relative humidity low and raise the inner surface temperature. However, it is essential to maintain at least a modest level of humidity inside the mask in order to avoid a dry throat.

The principle of condensation inside the mask is explained in this section. Particular emphasis is placed on factors that contribute to condensation as well as heat and mass transfer inside the mask. It is shown that thermodynamic laws can be used to calculate the condensation rate in the process of evaluating the performance of a CPAP mask.

6.3.1 Condensation Physics

There are two forms of condensation: film condensation and dropwise condensation. Initially, film condensation forms and subsequently dropwise condensation takes place. For film condensation, the condensate wets the surface and forms a liquid film on the surface, which slides down under the influence of gravity (Figure 6-5). The thickness of the liquid film (δ_f) increases in the flow direction as more vapors condense on the film.

Condensation occurs when water vapor is cooled below its saturation temperature as a result of heat transfer. The gas-vapor boundary layer forms next to the condensate layer, and the partial pressures of gas and vapor vary through the boundary layer. The buildup of non-condensable gas near the condensate film inhibits the diffusion of the vapor from the bulk mixture to the liquid film, and reduces the rate of mass and energy transfer. It is necessary to simultaneously solve the conservation equations of mass, momentum, and energy for both the condensate film and the vapor-gas boundary layer. In addition, the presence of air inside the mask acting as non-condensable gas makes this analysis even more complicated. Conservation of species may be introduced for this

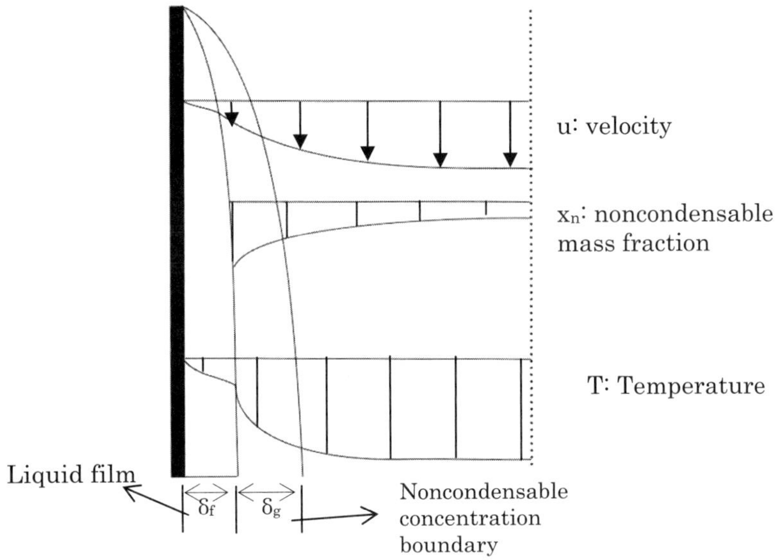

Figure 6-5. Schematic of boundary layer

instance. Computer solvers are usually introduced to solve the governing equations mentioned above. For a quantifying analysis, the condensation rate needs to be used. To simplify this analysis, the following assumptions are made:

1. For the liquid film, the flow is laminar with constant properties.
2. The heat resistance caused by the film is negligible as it contributes only 1% to 3% to the total heat resistance.
3. The shear stress at the liquid-vapor interface is assumed to be negligible.
4. The mask wall is considered as a vertical plate, and the film originates at the top of the plate and flows downward under the influence of gravity.
5. Gases inside the mask are assumed to be of a non-condensable nature.
6. For the entire mask use there is no significant change in the density of the air inside the mask.
7. The properties of water are calculated at the average temperature between the saturation temperature and the mask wall temperature.

6.3.2 Calculation of condensation rate

The heat flux is generally from the mask to the ambient surroundings, and it is due to the temperature difference between the inside and outside

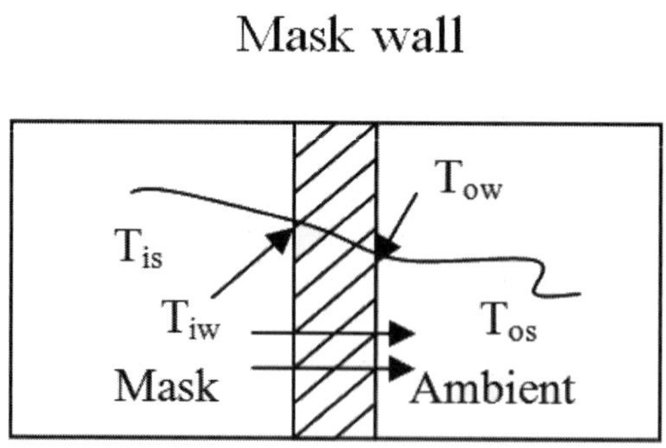

Figure 6-6. Mask heat transfer

of the mask (Figure 6-6). The thermal circuit consists of internal and external heat transfer films, in addition to the wall thermal resistance (Figure 6-6).

$$R_{tot} = R_{is} + R_{os} + R_w \tag{6-10}$$

with the inside film convective thermal resistance:

$$R_{is} = \frac{1}{h_{is}A_m} \tag{6-11}$$

the outside film convective thermal resistance:

$$R_{os} = \frac{1}{h_{os}A_m} \tag{6-12}$$

and the wall conduction resistance:

$$R_w = \frac{L_m}{kA_m} \tag{6-13}$$

where h_{is} and h_{os} are the convective heat transfer coefficients of the inside and outside wall surface of the mask, respectively.

Equation (6-10) may be written as:

$$R_{tot} = \frac{1}{h_{is}A_m} + \frac{1}{h_{os}A_m} + \frac{L_m}{kA_m} \tag{6-14}$$

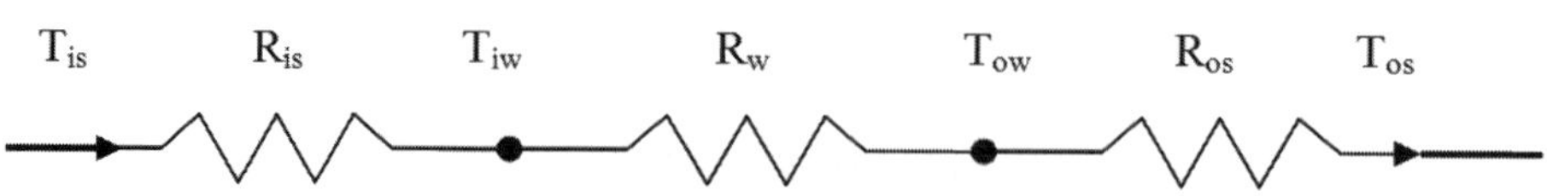

Figure 6-7. Thermal resistance model

At steady state, the heat flux from the mask to the ambient air can be written as:

$$Q_{tot} = \frac{T_{is} - T_{os}}{\dfrac{1}{h_{is}A_m} + \dfrac{1}{h_{os}A_m} + \dfrac{L_m}{kA_m}} \qquad (6-15)$$

It can be assumed that the heat transfer rates are equal at all points in the circuit. Therefore, the condensation rate can be determined by the convection heat transfer rate [8] inside the mask and expressed as:

$$\dot{m} = \frac{Q_{tot}}{h_{fg}{}^{*}} \qquad (6-16)$$

where Q_{tot} is the total heat transfer rate; and $h_{fg}{}^{*}$ is the modified latent heat of vaporization.

The modified latent heat of vaporization $h_{fg}{}^{*}$ can be obtained by:

$$h_{fg}^{*} = h_{fg} + 0.68C_{pl}(T_{sat} - T_s) \qquad (6-17)$$

where h_{fg} is the enthalpy of vaporization; C_{pl} is the specific heat of water at an average film temperature T_f; T_s is the wall surface temperature of the mask; and T_{sat} is the saturation temperature of water at specific pressure.

Substituting equation (6-15) and (6-17) into equation (6-16) yields

$$\dot{m} = \frac{\dfrac{T_{is} - T_{os}}{\dfrac{1}{h_{is}A_m} + \dfrac{1}{h_{os}A_m} + \dfrac{L_m}{kA_m}}}{h_{gf} + 0.68C_{pl}(T_{sat} - T_s)} \qquad (6-18)$$

Due to the parallel coexistence of gas and water inside the mask, the total condensation heat transfer coefficient inside the mask, $h_{is,}$ can be written as:

$$\frac{1}{h_{is}} = \frac{1}{h_{film}} + \frac{1}{h_{gas}} \qquad (6-19)$$

where h_{film} is the heat transfer coefficient for the condensation film; and h_{gas} is the heat transfer coefficient for gas.

Analysis of convective heat transfer problems is based on accurate knowledge of the heat transfer coefficient. The heat transfer coefficient is affected by many parameters that have been defined differently by various investigators. Experiments have demonstrated that the heat transfer convection coefficient can be correlated with flow velocity, fluid properties; and the geometry of the fluid surface [9]. When investigating forced convection problems, the fluid velocity is the dominant parameter. For the heat transfer coefficient of a water film, the velocity inside the mask is usually less than 3 m/s. This means that the Reynolds number, Re, is in the range of 30<Re<1800. Together with the fact that air density is much smaller than the water density, it can be concluded that wavy laminar flow represents the condensation inside the CPAP mask, hence h_{film} can be expressed as [10]:

$$h_{film} = \frac{R_{em}K_l}{1.08R_{em}^{1.22} - 5.2}\left(\frac{g}{V_l^2}\right)^{1/3} \qquad (6-20)$$

where K_l is thermal conductivity of water; V_l is the kinematic viscosity of water; g is the gravitational acceleration; and Rem is the local Reynolds number.

Radiative heat transfer is negligible for the temperature range of operation, so the heat transfer process consists of convective and conductive heat transfer only. As a result, the heat transfer coefficient for gas is:

$$h_{gas} = h_{convective} + h_{conductive} \qquad (6-21)$$

The conductive heat transfer coefficient $h_{conductive}$ can be expressed by [10]:

$$h_{conductive} = \frac{G_m(W_l - W_{bulk})\Delta h}{(1-W_l)(T_{sat} - T_f)} \qquad (6-22)$$

where W_l is the mass fraction of water; W_{bulk} is the bulk mass fraction; G_m is the mass transfer coefficient; and Δh is the change in specific enthalpy.

The convective heat transfer coefficient $h_{convective}$ can be obtained from the correlation between the friction factor and the Stanton number [10]:

$$St = \frac{h_{convective}}{\rho_g C_p \mu_g} = \frac{Cj}{2} Pr^{-1} \qquad (6-23)$$

with

$$\frac{Cj}{2} = 0.0296Rem^{-0.2} \qquad (6-24)$$

Combining the last two equations yields:

$$h_{convective} = 0.0592Rem - 0.2/Pr \qquad (6-25)$$

where Rem is the local Reynolds number; and Pr is the Prandtl number.

Equation (6-21) can then be rewritten as:

$$h_{gas} = 0.0592\,Re^{-0.2}/Pr + \frac{G_m(W_l - W_{bulk})\Delta h}{(1-W_l)(T_{sat} - T_f)} \qquad (6-26)$$

The total heat transfer coefficient can then be expressed as:

$$h_{is} = \frac{\left(0.0592 Re_m^{-0.2}/Pr + \frac{G_m(W_l - W_{bulk})\Delta h}{(1-W_l)(T_{sat}-T_f)}\right)\left(\frac{Re_m K_l}{1.08 Re_m^{1.22} - 5.2}\left(\frac{g}{v_l^2}\right)^{1/3}\right)}{0.0592 Re_m^{-0.2}/Pr + \frac{G_m(W_l - W_{bulk})\Delta h}{(1-W_l)(T_{sat}-T_f)} + \frac{\mathrm{Re}\, K_l}{1.08 Re_m^{1.22} - 5.2}\left(\frac{g}{v_l^2}\right)^{1/3}} \tag{6-27}$$

Applying these equations to a typical CPAP mask, Zhen [5] determined the condensation rate to be 4.5×10^{-6} g/s for a modified latent heat of vaporization, h_{fg}^*, of 2450 J/g. The total amount of condensation is estimated as 0.648 g for a patient wearing the mask over a period of 4 hours.

6.4 COMPUTATIONAL FLUID DYNAMIC (CFD) SIMULATIONS

Even though the average condensation rate can be calculated by the above model, it is still impossible to identify the exact location of condensation due to the temperature distribution inside the mask and the geometrical complexity of the mask. Numerical methods may be utilized in order to deal with the following issues:

- Temperature distribution: to identify the location that condensation most likely occurs, based on the fact that condensation will take place if the vapor temperature at that point is lower than its saturation temperature.
- Particle and trajectory plots: at the dead zone (stagnant area) where the flow vector is relatively small either during exhalation or inspiration. This information may be used to avoid condensation during product design.
- Optimize the position of the diffuser system to improve ventilation.
- Create a larger thermal resistance by increasing the wall thickness of the CPAP mask base or selecting materials with higher thermal conductivity.
- Parametric studies to determine orifice diameters capable of producing bias flow rates that maintain low CO_2 concentrations.
- Use of dynamic mesh techniques to study flow-driven deformation of the diaphragm and its effect on the bias flow rate.

Examples of such applications are shown in Figure 6-8 to Figure 6-10 [5], where CosmosFloWorks™ (an add-in program to the 3-D design package SolidWorks™) is used to run thermal and fluid dynamic simulations.

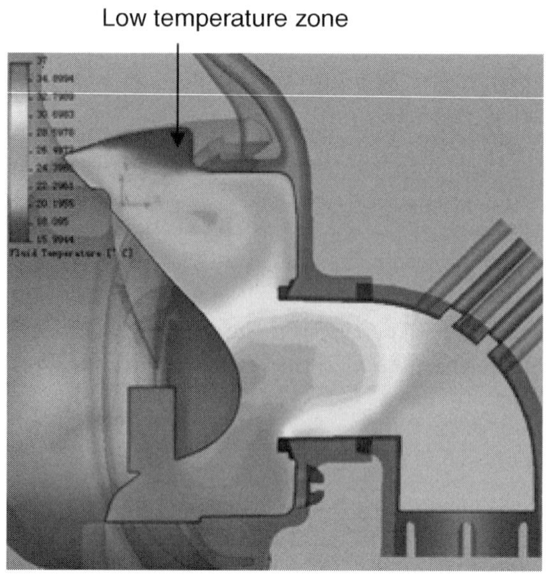

Figure 6-8. Temperature distribution for a CPAP mask [5]

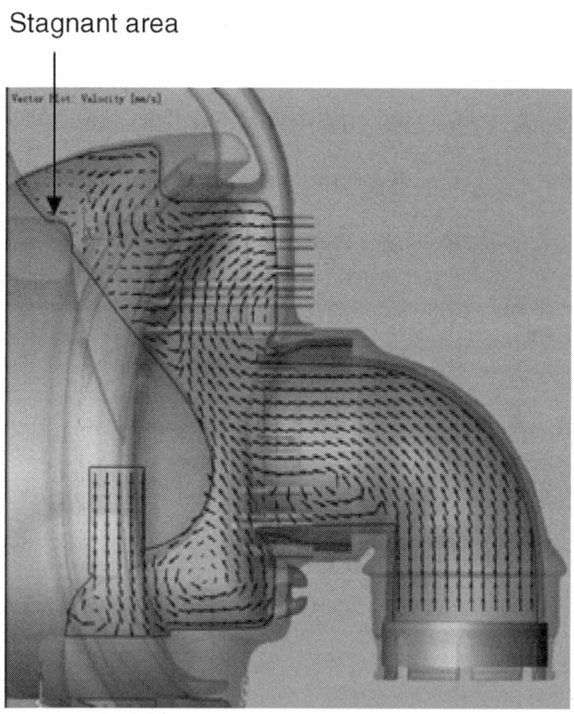

Figure 6-9. Velocity vectors predicting condensation location [5]

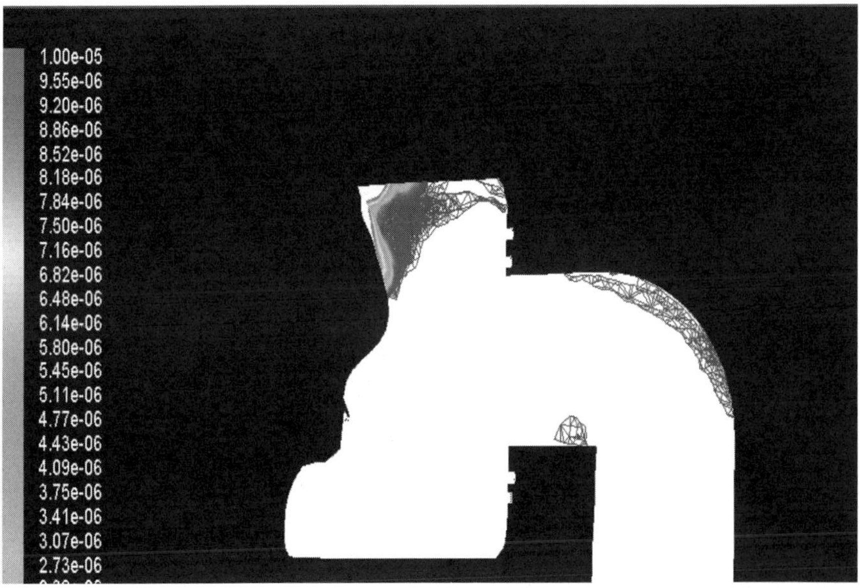

Figure 6-10. Contours of condensation rate (g/s) [5]

Temperature distribution plots (Figure 6-8) show the low temperature zones where condensation is most likely to occur. Velocity vector plots (Figure 6-9) indicate stagnant areas with relatively lower air velocity, which are also areas of condensation buildup.

In addition, user defined codes (UDF) can be used to customize multiphase fluid flow and heat transfer models as in Zhen [5], where C++ language was used to compute the condensation rate distribution within the mask under quiet breathing (Figure 6-10).

6.5 CLOSURE

This chapter deals with the issues faced in condensation and carbon dioxide concentration when designing CPAP masks. The manner in which the modeling process can be used in the selection of design parameters to minimize condensation and carbon dioxide buildup in the mask is illustrated. A combination of analytical as well as CFD approaches is used for this purpose.

REFERENCES

[1] Nakayama, H., Smith, C.A., Rodman, J.R., Skatrud, J.B., Dempsey, J.A., Effect of Ventilatory Drive on Carbon Dioxide Sensitivity Below Eupnea During Sleep. *Am J Respir Crit Care Med*, 2002. **165**(9): p. 1251–60.

[2] Klefbeck, B., Remmer, L., Weinberg, J., and Borg, J., A New Nasal Mask for Nocturnal Home Ventilation in Chronic Neuromuscular Disorders. *Scand J Rehabil Med*, 1993. **25**(1): p. 7–9.

[3] Schettino, G.P., Chatmongkolchart, S., Hess, D.R., and Kacmarek, R.M., Position of Exhalation Port and Mask Design Affect CO2 Rebreathing During Noninvasive Positive Pressure Ventilation. *Crit Care Med*, 2003. **31**(8): p. 2178–82.

[4] Patroniti, N., Foti, G., Manfio, A., Coppo, A., Bellani, G., and Pesenti, A., Head Helmet Versus Face Mask for Non-invasive Continuous Positive Airway Pressure: A Physiological Study. *Intensive Care Med*, 2003. **29**(10): p. 1680–87.

[5] Zhen, Z.F., CPAP Mask Thermo-Fluid Dynamics for Carbon Dioxide and Condensation Reduction, Master of Engineering thesis, 2005. Auckland University of Technology, Auckland, p. 111.

[6] Wu, D., *Analysis and Simulation of LSPC Hydraulic Systems*, 2003, University of Saskatchewan, Saskatoon.

[7] Merritt, H.E., *Hydraulic Control Systems*, 1967. John Wiley & Sons.

[8] Cengel, Y.A., *Heat Transfer: A Practical Approach*, 1998. McGraw-Hill.

[9] Stoeker, W.F. and Jones, J.W., *Refrigeration and Air Conditioning*, 1986. McGraw Hill.

[10] Azar, K. and Moffat, R.J., Heat Transfer Coefficient and Its Estimation in Electronic Enclosures, in *National Electronic Packaging and Production Conference*, 1991. Boston, MA, p. 361–72.

Part 2:

RESPIRATORY DISTRESS SYNDROME (RDS)

Chapter 7

BASIC PRINCIPLES AND CURRENT TREATMENTS

This chapter provides an introduction and overview of Respiratory Distress Syndrome (RDS). Current traditional surfactant and ventilation therapies are described, along with more current techniques that use pressure oscillations. In particular, the Bubble Continuous Positive Airway Pressure (CPAP) system is elaborated on, along with clinical studies from the literature that outline the benefits of its use to treat RDS.

7.1 RESPIRATORY DISTRESS SYNDROME (RDS)

The most common reason to initiate ventilation of a neonate (newborn infant) is respiratory failure. This can be caused by conditions that arise either from a failure of the central nervous system, or where there is a ventilation-perfusion mismatch caused by physiological disruptions. Conditions arising from the first type are apnea due to prematurity, intracranial hemorrhage, birth asphyxia, and drug overdose. In these cases, the neonate does not breathe because the respiratory drive is suppressed, and hence mechanical ventilation (MV) is absolutely necessary. In the second type, pulmonary gas exchange is inadequate to sustain required partial pressures of arterial carbon dioxide ($PaCO_2$) and oxygen (PaO_2). The inadequacy in gas exchange is caused by diseases stemming from physiological changes, inflammation and infection of membranes in the respiratory system, such as RDS, pneumonia, pneumothorax, diaphragmatic hernia, and tumors [1]. Of specific interest for this research is RDS (previously called hyaline membrane disease).

RDS is the most common respiratory illness to affect neonates. It remains the leading cause of infant mortality and morbidity. With the progress in technology, there are increasing options for providing quality respiratory ventilation for neonates. Irrespective of the type of respiratory ventilation, the goals of ventilation remain the same, namely to maintain adequate gas exchange in the lungs and reduce the Work of Breath (WOB) of the patient, while minimizing injury to the lungs and maintaining the highest level of patient comfort. The traditional method of respiratory ventilation has been mechanical ventilators. However, the use of such ventilators on delicate premature lungs causes many of the survivors of RDS to develop Bronchopulmonary Dysplasia (BPD) resulting from barotrauma [2-4]. Ventilation at low lung volumes also worsen lung injury due to the repetitive opening and closing of collapsed regions (atelectrauma) [5, 6]. A variety of other respiratory support techniques have been administered in an effort to reduce the possibility of overdistension of the airways and shear stresses on the epithelial walls, as is common in mechanical ventilation.

7.1.1 Pathophysiology

RDS is caused by insufficient surfactant production in the alveoli (air sacs) and underdeveloped lung structure [1, 7-9]. Surfactant and lung structure development can be explained in the context of gestational age with the aid of Figure 7-1 [1, 7]. Lung development is partitioned into five phases:

1. Embryonic phase (3 to 6 weeks)
2. Pseudoglandular phase (6 to 16 weeks)
3. Canalicular phase (16 to 26 weeks)
4. Saccular phase (26 to 36 weeks)
5. Alveolar phase (36 weeks to 3 years)

The expected date of delivery is calculated at 40 weeks of pregnancy. Normal pregnancy is considered to occur between 37 to 42 weeks. Infants born before 37 weeks of age are considered to be preterm, and infants are termed as neonates up to 28 days after birth.

Surfactant is produced by the alveolar type II cells in lamellar bodies. It performs the function of decreasing the surface tension forces at the air-liquid interface in the alveoli and is therefore a prerequisite to breathing. Once secreted by the lamellar bodies, the surfactant is transported to the air-liquid interface where it spreads as a monolayer and acts to reduce the surface tension. This process starts around week

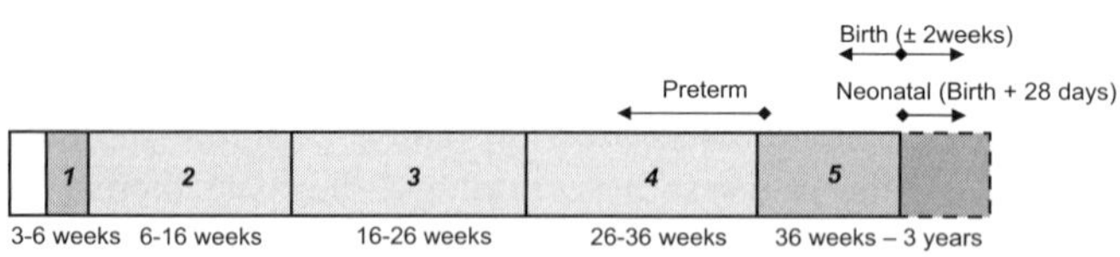

Figure 7-1. Human lung development with gestation

26 post-conception and is not yet fully completed in the saccular phase (26 to 36 weeks). Infants born in this period have lungs with insufficient surfactant and alveoli to facilitate adequate ventilation. A lack of surfactant in preterm infants means that the surface tension forces in their alveoli are much higher and act to decrease the surface area of the alveoli to such an extent that they collapse, marking the onset of RDS.

Traditional surfactant therapies and ventilation techniques have been used in neonatal intensive care units (NICUs) to treat RDS. These are discussed in Sections 7.1.2 and 7.1.3, respectively.

7.1.2 Surfactant Therapies

Natural surfactants that are currently used in the treatment of RDS are lipid extracts of bovine lung mince (Surfactant TA and Survanta), extracts of bovine lung washes (Infasurf, Alveofact, and BLES), and extracts of porcine lung mince (Curosurf).

Examples of synthetic surfactants are Exosurf and Pumactant. The main incentive toward their development is the high price of natural surfactant. They are usually highly simplified mixtures of phospholipids and do not contain the surfactant proteins that natural surfactants contain, which usually enhance the surface tension lowering ability of the surfactant. Surfaxin and Venticute contain additives that have surfactant protein-like properties. However, to date there is no clinical evidence to suggest which natural surfactant is superior and whether synthetic surfactants are superior to natural preparations [10, 11].

Surfactant treatments have shown to improve oxygenation and lung mechanics as well as lower the mean airway pressures and the percentage concentration of oxygen in the gas (fraction of inspired oxygen - FiO_2) delivered by ventilators to premature infants with RDS. Surfactant can be administered either prophylactically (within 10 minutes of birth), as an early treatment (within 2 hours of birth), or as a rescue treatment (when RDS has been established). Although there are no trials comparing prophylactic treatment with early treatment, clinical trials have been done to show that early treatment is definitely more effective than delaying treatment until RDS has been established [1, 10, 11].

7.1.3 Traditional Ventilation Therapies

It was not until the 1970s that the practice of neonatal mechanical ventilation advanced and dramatically improved the treatment of neonates with RDS. Traditional modes of mechanical ventilation include Intermittent Mandatory Ventilation (IMV) and Synchronized Intermittent Mandatory Ventilation (SIMV) with pressure and volume control modes. Early techniques of IMV functioned by taking over the role of the respiratory muscles by facilitating gas exchange. The ventilator could be pre-set to deliver "mechanical breaths" at regular breath cycles. The disadvantage was that infants often breathed asynchronously with the mechanical breaths, which led to inefficient gas exchange, gas trapping, and air leaks [12-14].

This non-synchronization between the infant and the ventilator led to the development of an improved type of ventilator, SIMV. This type of ventilator synchronized the mechanical breaths with the infant's spontaneous breath. In simpler terms, the ventilator looked for a spontaneous breath from the patient within a timing window each time it was supposed to cycle and would either start or delay the mechanical breaths if a spontaneous breath was detected [12, 13]. Although this synchronized the inspiratory process, the expiratory process was still subject to asynchrony.

Clinicians have the option within a ventilatory mode to choose between Pressure-Controlled Ventilation (PCV) and Volume-Controlled Ventilation (VCV). Controlling the applied pressure works such that if a consistent Peak Inspiratory Pressure (PIP) is set, the volume of air delivered to the patient would be dependent on the compliance of the lung. This meant that if the compliance was poor, the infant would receive a lower volume than required and if the compliance improved, the infant would receive a higher volume. Controlling the tidal volume, however, does not present much improvement of the undesirable possibility of generating high pressures in the lung. A reduced compliance, increased resistance, or active exhalation increases the risk of ventilator-induced lung injury such as BPD [12-14].

BPD is a type of lung injury in preterm infants brought on by too much oxygen and mechanical ventilation [2, 12, 15-17]. Mechanical ventilation not only causes damage and inflammation in the delicate premature lungs, but also impairs the lungs' ability to repair itself and develop further. Clinical investigations using mechanical ventilation performed on a number of species showed that lungs that were exposed to high levels of oxygen in an attempt to achieve higher levels of oxygen saturation in the blood developed significant persistent lung disease [17]. Studies on preterm animals also showed that mechanical ventilation damaged lungs by causing an inflammatory response [16, 18, 19].

Due to the high risks involved with mechanical ventilation, other "gentler" techniques have been developed such as High-Frequency Ventilation (HFV), Biologically Variable Ventilation (BVV), and CPAP to avoid neonates from progressing to respiratory failure. HFV is characterized by high frequency rates up to 15 Hz at volumes less than the dead space of the lung, while BVV uses a computer controller to deliver typical physiological variations in tidal volume and breath rate. These methods along with the traditional method of CPAP and the Bubble CPAP System, which is a modified form of traditional CPAP that also produces pressure oscillations, is discussed in further detail in Section 7.2.

7.2 VENTILATION TECHNIQUES USING PRESSURE OSCILLATIONS

The use of pressure oscillations in ventilation before the introduction of Bubble CPAP was not entirely unknown. This section presents a review of the literature focusing on the description of the ventilation techniques that use pressure oscillations, their clinical benefits, and proposed mechanisms of improvement.

7.2.1 High Frequency Ventilation (HFV)

HFV was a radical departure from mechanical ventilation in that it delivered gas at small tidal volumes (less than the dead space of the lung) at frequencies up to 15 Hz. The pulses of small gas volumes at rapid rates created lower pressures in the alveoli, decreasing the incidence of lung tissue injury [20-23]. It has been suggested that the vibratory or pulsing nature of the airflow causes a "sloshing motion" of air in the lungs, known as pendelluft, and that this feature of HFV may offer better gas transport to the respiratory zone of the lung [24, 25]. Clinical results [26, 27] have shown that early, exclusive use of HFV decreases the incidence of BPD in premature infants with RDS when compared to mechanical ventilation. Infants also required a much shorter period on ventilator support.

A number of mechanisms of gas transport during HFV have been suggested. During normal breathing frequencies, bulk convection and molecular diffusion take place. These mechanisms also occur during HFV but other mechanisms have also been suggested. Chang [24] proposed that the following modes of gas transport are collectively responsible during HFV:

Direct alveolar ventilation - Alveoli that lie proximal to the trachea still receive direct ventilation. Even though the tidal volumes are small, as long as they are above a certain limit, some alveoli will receive fresh gas with every inspiration.

Pendelluft - When neighboring regions in the lung are different in compliance, resistance, and time constants of inflation and deflation, it leads to "fast" units that fill faster and more easily ((Figure 7-2(a)), and "slow" units that may still be in the process of inhalation when the fast units are exhaling (Figure 7-2(b)). During high velocity flow this phenomenon is magnified and the neighboring units mutually exchange gas in an effect known as pendelluft. As a result, there is a more homogeneous mixing of gas, allowing the use of smaller volumes of gas to reach more alveoli and, as a result, decrease the amount of tidal volume required for respiration.

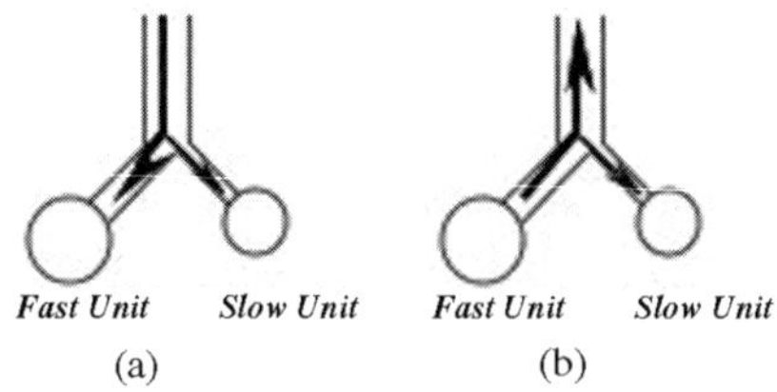

Figure 7-2. Pendelluft phenomenon showing filling and emptying of units

Convective Gas Transport - During inspiration the velocity profile of the gas is parabolic (Figure 7-3(b)), but during expiration the velocity profile is flatter (Figure 7-3(c)). The resulting displacement of a particle of gas that was situated at the center of the airway at the start of inspiration (Figure 7-3(a)) is now situated to the right (Figure 7-3(d)) (i.e., working its way down the tracheo-bronchial tree to the alveoli) and the gas particles near the walls are situated to the left of their original position.

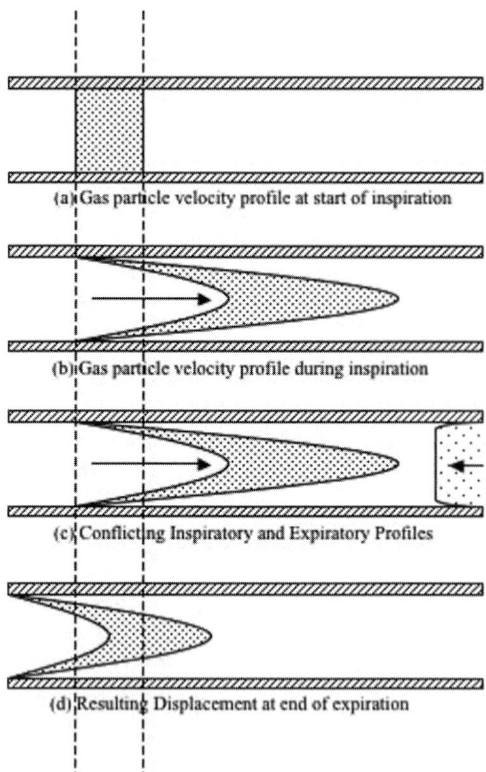

Figure 7-3. Velocity profiles during convective gas transport

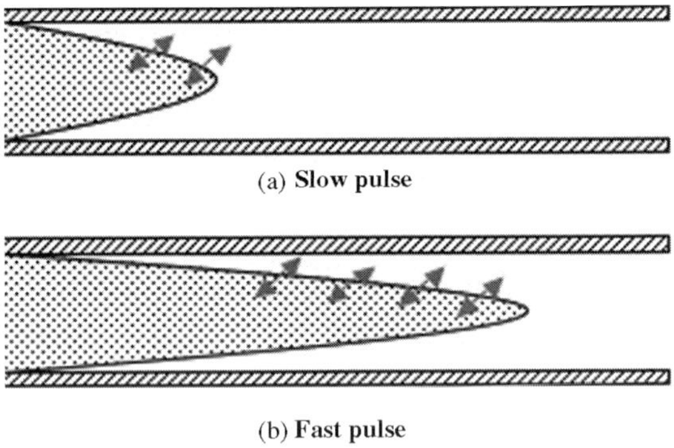

Figure 7-4. Facilitated diffusion during HFV

Facilitated diffusion - The fast pulses of low volumes in HFV move down the airways with larger axial spikes (Figure 7-4(b)) than slower pulses (Figure 7-4(a)), which create a larger boundary for lateral diffusion of oxygen and carbon dioxide in laminar flow.

Lateral diffusion can also occur in turbulent flow and at bifurcations due to eddies. Thus, it is said that diffusion is facilitated in these cases.

Molecular Diffusion - This refers to the molecular diffusion of respiratory gases at the alveolar-capillary membrane. This mechanism always exists as along as gas exists there at a temperature above absolute zero, and hence is not an HFV-specific mechanism. Molecular diffusion of oxygen and carbon dioxide will occur across the alveolar-capillary membrane to maintain an equilibrium between partial pressures of these gases.

De Jong [28] also suggested that another factor of importance for HFV is surfactant efficiency. The fact that HFV has lower pressures may mean that they do not "disturb" the critical alveoli (which have a relatively low surfactant concentration) and so they will not collapse.

Although all six modes of gas transport discussed may exist during HFV, it is possible that certain modes are more dominant in certain regions of the respiratory system. It has been suggested that direct ventilation and facilitated diffusion dominate ventilation in the trachea, while pendelluft or convective gas transport dominate in the medium-size airways. Smaller airways are ventilated by pendelluft and alveoli by molecular diffusion. There are many variants of the HFV technique, but they all contain three basic elements: a high pressure flow generator, a valve for flow interruption, and a breathing circuit to be connected to the patient. Variants include high-frequency jet ventilation (HFJV), high-frequency flow interruption (HFFI), high-frequency (push-pull) oscillation (HFO), high-frequency positive pressure ventilation (HFPPV), and high-frequency percussive ventilation (HFPV).

7.2.2 Biologically Variable Ventilation (BVV)

Biologically variable ventilation or "noisy ventilation" has been clinically shown to have benefits as well. BVV uses a computer controller to mimic the normal variability in a spontaneously breathing lung by producing random variations in tidal volume and breath rate. Studies on porcine [29, 30] and rodent [31] models showed that such techniques improve the oxygenation of arterial blood and have enhanced the performance of mechanical ventilators. Mathematical models [32] that were developed also suggest that mechanical ventilation accompanied by randomly varying breath patterns improved alveolar recruitment by opening collapsed alveoli and increasing the net lung volume without causing increases in mean airway pressures.

The mechanisms of alveolar recruitment for this technique are also not fully understood, although theories do exist on the mechanisms of gas transport. These are mostly associated with the benefits due to the better mixing of gases in noisy ventilation [24, 25, 33].

Various authors suggest that noisy ventilation (like BVV and Bubble CPAP) is an example of stochastic resonance [21, 30, 32, 34]. Studies on small animals [30, 31] have shown that respiratory support systems can optimize lung recruitment by tuning parameters such as the timing and amplitude of the pressure fluctuations. Whether this is applicable to larger animals and humans remains to be proven.

7.2.3 Continuous Positive Airway Pressure (CPAP) With Pressure Oscillations

Nasal Continuous Positive Airway Pressure (nCPAP) is a non-invasive type of respiratory support in comparison to endotracheal ventilation. It applies a continuous positive pressure to the alveoli (through nasal prongs or tubes) throughout the respiratory cycle and has been increasingly used in hospitals to treat neonates with RDS [35, 36]. The positive pressure applied to the lung is created by a variable resistance at exhalation. It produces a more regular breathing pattern when compared to mechanical ventilation since it allows the infant to breathe spontaneously. The continuous distending pressure provided by nCPAP increases lung volume and promotes better gas exchange in the alveoli by keeping them open [8, 12]. Studies have shown that nCPAP reduced the need for mechanical ventilation in neonates with moderate RDS and proved to be an adequate form of ventilation by improving oxygenation without causing any additional harmful side effects [37-40]

The Bubble CPAP System uses a water column rather than a variable resistor to produce the required CPAP to the alveoli. The bubbles produced in the CPAP bottle as the air leaves the system result in pressure oscillations (reported to be between 15 and 30 Hz [41]) in addition to the mean pressure. There has been some evidence based on studies of infants between 750 and 2500 g birth weight that using Bubble CPAP decreases the respiratory rate and minute ventilation in neonates with RDS without decreasing alveolar ventilation [41], meaning that the infant has to perform less muscle work to achieve adequate respiration. It was proposed that Bubble CPAP might facilitate better gas exchange in the lung, which may be caused by mechanisms seen in HFV.

Hospital and clinical studies have identified several benefits of Bubble CPAP that make it a feasible device for managing RDS in neonates. Hospital studies on preterm and extremely low birth weight infants concluded that the use of Bubble CPAP reduces the possibility of lung injury by reducing the need and number of days required for mechanical ventilation [35, 42, 43]. Studies also showed that hospitals that used Bubble CPAP to a greater extent on preterm infants with RDS reported a significantly lower rate of BPD than hospitals that did not [42, 44, 45].

A notable study by Pillow et al. [46] on preterm lambs showed that (in comparison to constant pressure CPAP) Bubble CPAP improved arterial oxygen levels (due to the improved gas exchange offered by the pressure oscillations), stabilized lung volumes at low pressure, and enhanced lung mechanics (by increasing compliance and Functional Residual Capacity (FRC) and decreasing airway resistance).

Studies on preterm lambs have also shown that Bubble CPAP improves the compliance of the lung by preventing repetitive inflammatory stresses on the preterm lung and preserving surfactant function better than mechanical ventilation [47]. It has also been speculated that the noisy pressure signal may also promote surfactant secretion in the lung [48].

The improvements noted in ventilatory parameters during Bubble CPAP could be due to a number of physiological, chemical, and mechanical mechanisms. These include the avoidance of aggressive initiation of ventilation with high tidal volumes and inadvertent hyperventilation of the lung [43, 47], similar to those seen in HFV [41] and that of stochastic resonance resulting from the superimposed noisy pressure signal from the bubbling action [46]. However, the relative contributions of the different proposed mechanisms are yet to be established.

The essence of stochastic resonance in relation to the Bubble CPAP System can be explained as follows. When "noise" is added to the input in a non-linear system (like the lung), the response is first improved. However, it is possible that if the timing or the pressure amplitude of the noise is increased further it can have a detrimental effect. This suggests that noise can be tuned in such a way as to provide optimal ventilation [31, 32]. This improvement has been illustrated in terms of the net volume recruited due to the non-linearity of the pressure-volume curves of the lung. However, the stochastic resonance effect due to the overall mechanical response of the respiratory system is yet to be determined, and is of interest to this research.

To date no clinical studies have ventured so far as to determine the optimum amplitude and frequencies of pressure oscillations in the treatment of RDS. Some analytical studies [49, 50] demonstrate the ability of using the Bubble CPAP System to optimize the amplitudes and frequencies of pressure oscillations produced by the system, but these remain to be validated by clinical studies.

7.3 CLOSURE

The background and pathophysiology of RDS is given in this chapter. Traditional ventilation therapies to combat RDS are described along with newer techniques that utilize pressure oscillations and noisy signals.

REFERENCES

[1] Goldsmith, J.P. and Karotkin, E.H., Assisted Ventilation of the Neonate, 2003. Saunders, Philadelphia.
[2] Parker, J.C., Hernandez, L.A., and Peevy, K.J., Mechanisms of Ventilator-Induced Lung Injury. *Crit Care Med*, 1993. **21**: p. 131–43.
[3] Dreyfuss, D. and Saumon, G. Ventilator-Induced Lung Injury: Lessons From Experimental Studies. *Am J Respir Crit Care Med*, 1998. **157**: p. 294–323.
[4] Pierson, D.J., Alveolar Rupture During Mechanical Ventilatiob: Role of PEEP, Peak Airway Pressure, and Distending Volume. *Respir Care*, 1988. **33**: p. 472–86.
[5] Robertson, B., Batenburg, J.J., and Van Golde, L.M., Pulmonary Surfactant, 1994. Elsevier, Amsterdam.
[6] Muscedere, J.G., et al., Tidal Ventilation at Low Airway Pressures Can Augment Lung Injury. *Am J Respir Crit Care Med*, 1994. **149**(5): p. 1327–34.
[7] Gray, H., Gray's Anatomy of the Human Body, 2000. Lea and Febiger, Philadelphia.
[8] Polin, R.A. and Fox, W.W., Fetal and Neonatal Physiology, 2nd Ed. 1997. WB Saunders Co., Philadelphia.
[9] Avery, M.E. and Mead, J., Surface Properties in Relation to Atelectasis and Hyaline Membrane Disease. *A.M.A J Dis Child*, 1959. **97**: p. 517–23.
[10] Been, J.V. and Zimmerman, L.J.I., What's New in Surfactant? Eur J Paediatric, 2007. **166**: p. 889–99.
[11] Morley, C. and Davis, P., Surfactant Treatment for Premature Lung Disorders: A Review of Best Practices in 2002. *Paediatric Respiratory Reviews*, 2004. **5**(Suppl A): p. S299–S304.
[12] Donn, S.M. and Sinha, S.K., Invasive and Noninvasive Neonatal Ventilation. *Respir Care*, 2003. **48**: p. 426–41.
[13] Greenough, A. and Sharma, A., What is New in Ventilation Strategies for the Neonate? *Eur J Pedriatr*, 2007. **166**: p. 991–96.
[14] Schreiner, R.L. and Kisling, J.A., Practical Neonatal Respiratory Care, 1982. Raven Press, New York.
[15] Bezzant, T.B. and Mortensen, J.D., Risks and Hazards of Mechanical Ventilation: A Collective Review of Published Literature. *Disease-a-Month*, 1994. **40**: p. 581–640.
[16] Jobe, A.H. and Bancalari, E., Bronchopulmonary Dysplasia. *Am J Respir Crit Care Med*, 2001. **163**: p. 1723–29.

[17] Slutsky, A.S. and Tremblay, L.N., Multiple System Organ Failure. Is Mechanical Ventilation a Contributing Factor? *Am J Respir Crit Care Med*, 1998. **157**: p. 1721–25.
[18] Coalson, J.J., Winter, V., and deLemos, R.A., Decreased Alveolarisation in Baboon Survivors With Bronchopulmonary Dysplasia. *Am J Respir Crit Care Med*, 1995. **152**: p. 640–46.
[19] Naik, A., et al., Effects of Different Styles of Ventilation on Cytokine Expression in Preterm Lamb Lung. *Paediatric Respiratory Reviews*, 2000. **47**: p. 370A.
[20] Kesler, M. and Durand, D.J., Neonatal High-Frequency Ventilation. Past, Present and Future. *Clinical Perinatol*, 2001. **28**(3): p. 579–607.
[21] Owen, M.R. and Lewis, M.A., The Mechanics of Lung Tissue Under High-Frequency Ventilation. *SIAM J on Appl Math*, 2001. **61**(5): p. 1731–61.
[22] Ritacca, F.V. and Stewart, T.E., Clinical Review: High Frequency Osillatory Ventilation in Adults — A Review of the Literature and Practical Applications. *Crit Care*, 2003. **7**: p. 385–90.
[23] Wheeler, H.J., Nokes, L.D.M., and Powell, T., A Review of High Frequency Oscillation Ventilation in the Neonate. *J of MedEngrg and Technol*, 2007. **31**(5): p. 367–74.
[24] Chang, H.K., Mechanisms of Gas Transport During Ventilation by High Frequency Oscillation. *J Appl Physiol*, 1984. **56**(3): p. 553–63.
[25] High, K.C., Ultham, J.S., and Karl, S.R., Mechanically Induced Pendelluft Flow in a Model Airway Bifurcation During High Frequency Oscillation. *Transactions of the ASME*, 1991. **113**: p. 342–47.
[26] Courtney, S.E., et al., High Frequency Oscillatory Ventilation Versus Conventional Mechanical Ventilation for Very Low Birth Weight Infants. *Pediatrics*, 2002. **347**: p. 643–52.
[27] Rimensberger, P.C., et al., First Intention High Frequency Oscillation With Early Lung Volume Optimisation Improves Pulmonary Outcome in Low Birth Weight Infants With Respiratory Distress Syndrome. *Pediatrics*, 2000. **105**: p. 1202–08.
[28] De Jongh, F., Ventilation Modelling of the Human Lung, in Faculty of Aerospace Engineering, 1995. Delft University of Technology, Delft. p. 197.
[29] Mutch, W.A.C., et al., Biologically Variable or Naturally Noisy Mechanical Ventilation Recruits Atelectic Lung. *Am J Respir Crit Care Med*, 2000. **162**: p. 319–23.
[30] Mutch, W.A.C., et al., BVV Increases Arterial Oxygenation Over That Seen With Positive End-Expiratory Pressure Alone in a Porcine Model of Acute Rspiratory Distress Syndrome. *Crit Care Med*, 2000. **28**(7): p. 2457–63.
[31] Arold, S.P., et al., Variable Tidal Volume Ventilation Improves Lung Mechanics and Gas Exchange in a Rodent Model of Acute Lung Injury. *Am J Respir Crit Care Med*, 2002. **165**: p. 366–71.
[32] Suki, B., et al., Life Support System Benefits From Noise. *Nature*, 1998. **393**: p. 127–28.
[33] Otis, A.B., et al., Mechanical Factors in Distribution of Pulmonary Ventilation. *J Appl Physiol*, 1956. **8**: p. 427–43.
[34] Mutch, W.A.C, Harms, S. Lefevre, G.R., Graham, M.R., Girling, L.G., Kowalski, S.E., BVV Increases Arterial Oxygenation Over That Seen With Positive End-Expiratory Pressure Alone in a Porcine Model of Acute Respiratory Distress |Syndrome. *Crit Care Med*, 2000. **28**(7): p. 2457–63.

[35] Gitterman, M.K., et al., Early Nasal Continuous Positive Airway Pressure Treatment Reduces the Need for Intubation in Very Low Birth Weight Infants. *Eur J Pedriatr*, 1997. **156**: p. 384–88.

[36] Locke, R., Greenspan, J.S., and Shaffer, T.H., Effect of Nasal CPAP on Thoracoabdominal Motion in Neonates With Respiratory Insufficiency. *Pediatric Pulmonology*, 1991. **11**(3): p. 259–64.

[37] De Klerk, A.M. and De Klerk, R.K., Use of Continuous Positive Airways Pressure in Preterm Infants: Comments and Experience From New Zealand. *Pediatrics*, 2001. **108**(3): p. 761–63.

[38] Gitterman, M.K., Fusch, C., Gitterman, A.R., Regazonni, B.M., and Moessinger, A.C., Early Nasal Continuous Positive Airway Pressure Treatment Reduces the Need for Intubation in Very Low Birth Weight Infants. *Eur J Pedriatr*, 1997. **156**: p. 384–88.

[39] Mazzella, M., Bellini, C., Caleve, M.G., Campone, Massocco, F., Mezzano, D., Zullino, E., Scopesi, F., Arioni, C., Bonaci, W., and Serra, G., A Randomised Control Study Comparing the Infant Flow Driver With Nasal Continuous Positive Airway Pressure in Preterm Infants. *Arch Dis Child Fetal Neonatal*, 2001. **35**: p. F86–90.

[40] Verder, H., et al., Nasal Continuous Positive Airway Pressure and Early Surfactant Therapy for Respiratory Distress Syndrome in Newborns of Less than 30 Weeks' Gestation. *Pediatrics*, 1999. **103**(2): p. E24.

[41] Lee, K.S., et al., A Comparison of Underwater Bubble Continuous Positive Airway Pressure With Ventilator-Derived Continuous Positive Airway Pressure in Premature Neonates Ready for Extubation. *Biology of the Neonate*, 1998. **73**(69): p. 69–75.

[42] De Klerk, A.M. and De Klerk, R.K., Nasal Positive Airway Pressure and Outcomes of Preterm Infants. *J Pediatr Child Health*, 2001. **37**: p. 161–67.

[43] Narendran, V., et al., Early Bubble CPAP and Outcomes in ELBW Preterm Infants. *J Perinatology*, 2003. **23**(3): p. 195–9.

[44] Avery, M.E., Tooley, W., and Keller, J.B., Is Chronic Lung Disease in Low Birth Weight Infants Preventable? A Survey of Eight Centres. *Pediatrics*, 1987. **79**(1): p. 26–29.

[45] Van Marter, L.J., et al., Do Clinical Markers of Barotrauma and Oxygen Toxicity Explain Interhospital Variation in Rates of Chronic Lung Disease? *Pediatrics*, 2000. **105**(6): p. 1194–1201.

[46] Pillow, J., et al., Bubble Continuous Positive Airway Pressure Enhances Lung Volume and Gas Exchange in Preterm Lambs. *Am J Respir Crit Care Med*, 2007. **176**: p. 63–69.

[47] Jobe, A.H., et al., Decreased Indicators of Lung Injury with Continuous Positive Expiratory Pressure in Preterm Lambs. *Pediatric Res*, 2002. **52**(3).

[48] Arold, S.P., et al., Variable Ventilation Induces Endogenuous Surfactant Release in Normal Guinea Pigs. *Am J Physiol Lung Cell Mol Physiol*, 2006. **285**: p. L370–80.

[49] Manilal, P., The Effect of Pressure Oscillations on Neonatal Breathing, Master of Engineering Thesis in Diagnostics and Control Research Centre, 2004. Auckland University of Technology, Auckland. p. 134.

[50] Manilal, P., Al-Jumaily, A., and Prime, N., The Effect of Pressure Oscillations on Neonatal Breathing. 2004 ASME International Mechanical Engineering Congress & Exposition, November 13–19, 2004. Anaheim, California.

Chapter 8

MODELING OF BUBBLE CPAP

This chapter provides a description of the various components of the Bubble Continuous Positive Airway Pressure (CPAP) System before embarking on a lumped parameter modeling approach where basic laws of physics and empirical relationships are applied to generate mathematical models of individual components. A description of how to create an overall computational model of the system in Simulink™ within the Matlab™ environment is presented. The process of validating the model with experimental data is elaborated on with the end result being a model that can be used for Bubble CPAP performance assessments.

8.1 PRINCIPLES OF OPERATION AND SYSTEM COMPONENTS

The Bubble CPAP System is designed to offer respiratory support to spontaneously breathing neonates suffering from Respiratory Distress Syndrome (RDS). It applies a mean CPAP accompanied by pressure oscillations to the airways and alveoli throughout the respiratory cycle. This maintains a degree of lung inflation during expiration, thus preventing lung collapse and making it easier for the neonate to breathe since a partially inflated alveolus is easier to expand than a fully collapsed one.

Pioneering work underpinning the Bubble CPAP System focused on trying to provide respiratory support to neonates with RDS to prevent them from progressing to respiratory failure. The early system (Figure 8-1) consisted of a humidifier, a circuit for gas flow, a nasal prong to connect the circuit to the infant's airway, and a water-filled bottle into which the distal end of the expiratory tubing is immersed to create a positive pressure in the circuit [1].

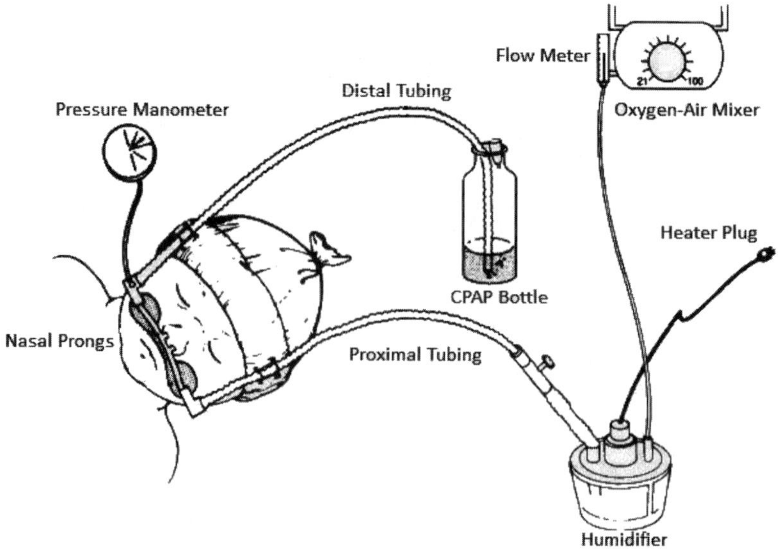

Figure 8-1. Initial bubble CPAP as used by Columbia Presbyterian Medical Centre [Reproduced with permission from Aly [1]]

The Bubble CPAP System operates under the same principles, but has been improved with features that offer more accuracy in maintaining required mean pressures and flows, as well as additional features that consider patient comfort. The system (Figure 8-2) includes a delivery system and a patient interface. The delivery system consists of a humidification chamber, a single-heated breathing circuit, CPAP generator, and pressure manifold. The patient interface consists of the nasal tubing, nasal prongs, and infant bonnet. Headgear may be used in place of the bonnet and chin straps (not shown) may also be added to the patient interface to optimize the effect of Bubble CPAP. The individual components (shown as they would appear in operation in Figure 8-2) are briefly described as follows.

8.1.1 Humidification Chamber

The chamber is the source of the humidity required by the neonate. Sterile water is fed into the chamber from a flexible bag. The water level is controlled by a dual float mechanism that prevents the chamber from flooding and provides a closed system and a constant mean CPAP pressure.

8.1.2 Single-Heated Breathing Circuit

The flexible breathing circuit (consisting of the inspiratory and expiratory lines) links the flow source, humidification chamber, patient interface, and CPAP generator. The inspiratory line connects the humidifier

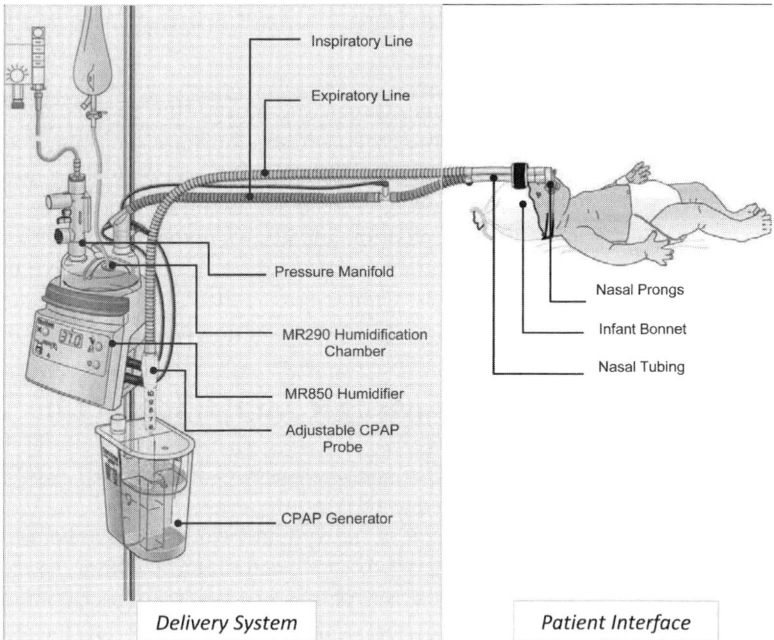

Figure 8-2. Bubble CPAP system components [Courtesy of Fisher & Paykel Healthcare Ltd]

to the patient interface and the transparent expiratory line connects the patient interface to the CPAP generator.

8.1.3 Pressure Manifold

The pressure manifold is a pressure relief mechanism situated upstream of the neonate that limits the maximum pressure in the system (typically around 17 cm H_2O at a flow rate of 8 L/min) in the event of an occlusion in the delivery system. It may also have measurement ports for pressure and air/oxygen analysis.

8.1.4 CPAP Generator

The CPAP generator is an innovative version of the early system of Bubble CPAP used at the Columbia Presbyterian Medical Center since 1974. Either lowering or raising the adjustable probe in the water container creates the required level of positive pressure in the circuit. Achievable mean pressures range from 3 to 10 cm H_2O. Excess water spills out into an overflow container ensuring that the mean CPAP pressure is constant. As air enters the water through the CPAP probe, it creates bubbles, which in turn create pressure oscillations about a mean CPAP level.

8.1.5 Patient Interface - Nasal Tubing, Nasal Prongs, and Infant Bonnet

The nasal tubing directs the air into the neonate and allows a balanced flow into the nares. To address the variety of nare diameters and septum gaps, nasal prongs of different sizes can be attached to the end of the nasal tubing. The specially designed infant bonnet allows for the nasal tubing to be fixed in position and allows repositioning of the nasal prongs with the infant's movements. Headgear as an alternative to the infant bonnet is also available. Chin straps are also available to prevent excessive leaks from the mouth, thereby preventing significant pressure loss.

8.2 LUMPED PARAMETER MODELING OF COMPONENTS

Each component of the system (with the exception of the pressure manifold) can be modeled as a separate control volume, as denoted in Figure 8-3. The physical characteristics and geometry of each component can be used to determine the correct values of the parameters and the physical relationships. Conservation laws of physics, coupled with fluid flow equations, are used to develop differential equations for each component of the system. Attempts are made throughout the modeling process to define elements as being pure and ideal where possible, since the model developed here serves as a building block to model a more real device more accurately in the future. Hence,

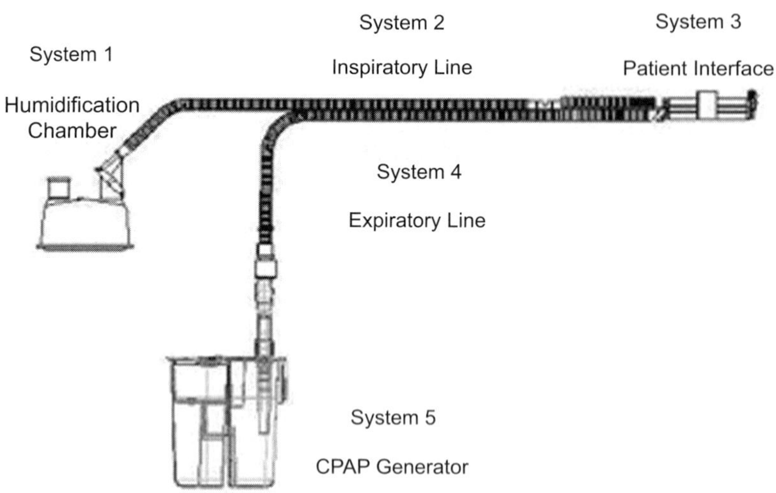

Figure 8-3. Control volumes in the bubble CPAP system for mathematical modeling

certain parameters such as the flow restrictions and shock factors at connections are ignored and descriptions of component resistances and capacitances tend toward more "unadulterated" system elements.

8.2.1 Humidification Chamber

Assumptions and Simplifications: The humidification chamber is modeled here as a reservoir with rigid boundaries. For simple introductory analyses covered in this chapter, where the effects of humidity are neglected and hence any changes in air properties due to temperature and phase changes can be ignored. The predominant dynamic effect of the humidification chamber is a function of its volume and so it acts as a pure capacitive element.

Derivation: Figure 8-4 shows the humidification chamber with internal pressure (P_H), mass inflow rate ($\dot{m}_{in}$), the mass outflow rate ($\dot{m}_{tube}$) and internal mass (M_H). Applying the conservation of mass to the control volume gives the change in mass of air in the chamber as:

$$\Delta M_H = m_{in} - m_{tube} \tag{8 – 1}$$

For a time-varying system

$$\frac{dM_H}{dt} = \frac{d}{dt}(m_{in} - m_{tube}) = \dot{m}_{in} - \dot{m}_{tube} \tag{8 – 2}$$

Because temperature and phase changes are ignored, as discussed earlier, the capacitance C_H and pressure P_H of the humidification chamber are determined by the following equation of state:

$$P_H V_H = M_H R_a T_H \tag{8 – 3}$$

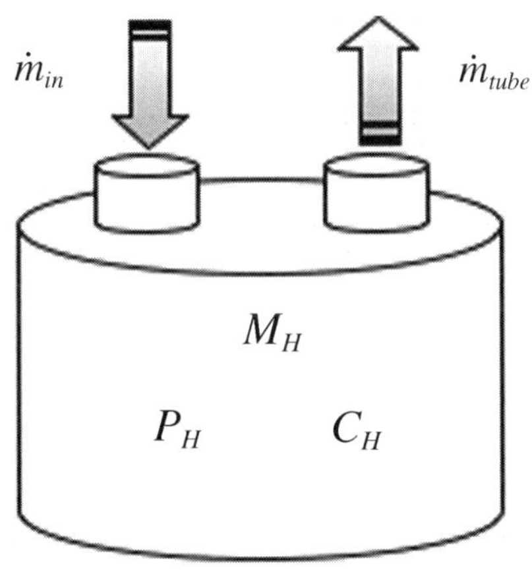

Figure 8-4. Modeling of the humidification chamber

where V_H and T_H are the volume and temperature of the mass of air in the chamber, respectively; and R_a is the gas constant of air. Rearranging the equation gives:

$$M_H = \frac{V_H}{R_a T_H} P_H \tag{8-4}$$

$\frac{V_H}{R_a T_H}$ is actually the capacitance (C_H) of the chamber, such that equation (8-4) becomes

$$M_H = C_H P_H \tag{8-5}$$

Substituting equation (8-5) into equation (8-2) yields the final equation for the chamber as:

$$\dot{m}_{in} - \dot{m}_{tube} = C_H \frac{dP_H}{dt} \tag{8-6}$$

Simulation Model: Figure 8-5 shows the model of the humidification chamber subsystem. The mass flows, $\dot{m}_{in}$ and $\dot{m}_{tube}$, are inputs, with the humidifier pressure, P_H, as the output. P_H then functions as one of the inputs into the inspiratory line subsystem.

8.2.2 The Inspiratory Line

Assumptions and Simplifications: The inspiratory line is a corrugated tube made of linear low-density polypropylene. It is often desirable to model fluid flow and pressure drops in a tube with Bernoulli's Equation. However, in situations such as the current one, it proves difficult to define parameters such as the Reynolds number and friction factor for such a tube. The problem is also compounded with the longitudinally varying

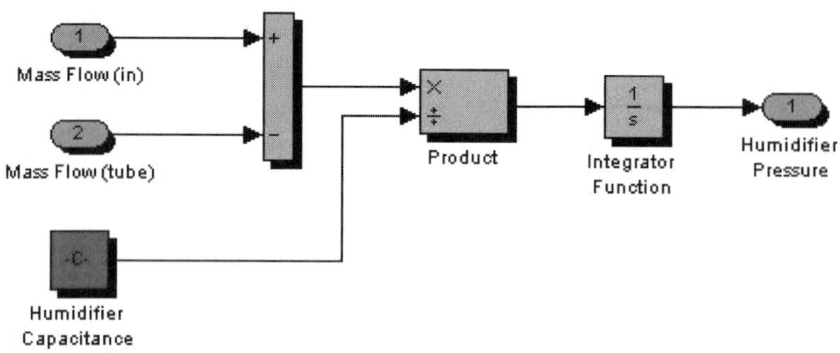

Figure 8-5. Humidification chamber subsystem

cross-sectional area of the tube, making it difficult and time-consuming to explore such methods. Since one of the features of lumped parameter modeling is the regular use of experimentally determined coefficients and relationships, the non-linear resistance in the inspiratory tube (R_{tube}) is defined by empirical methods.

Derivation: The resistance of the tube is dependent on the mass flow rate through it ($\dot{m}_{tube}$). When a fluid is forced through a tube at a constant flow rate, a pressure difference (as in Figure 8-6) related to that flow rate must be exerted to maintain that flow. Thus, it is possible to express the equation for the mass flow rate through the inspiratory line as follows:

$$\dot{m}_{tube} = \frac{P_H - P_{interface}}{R_{tube}} \qquad (8-7)$$

$P_{interface}$ is the pressure at the end of the inspiratory line, which is in fact the pressure at the patient interface, and $R_{tube} = f(\dot{m}_{tube})$.

To obtain the empirical relationship between R_{tube} and $\dot{m}_{tube}$, the static pressure drop across the inspiratory line needs to be measured for different mass flow rates from pressure taps at the beginning and end of the tube. This pressure drop $[(\Delta P = P_H - P_{interface})]$ has been previously measured by Manilal-Reddy and Al-Jumaily [2] for this particular system (as seen in Figure 8-7) and expressed as:

$$\Delta P = 2 \times 10^9 \dot{m}_{tube}^2 + 214329\, \dot{m}_{tube} + 0.9082 \qquad (8-8)$$

Combining equations (8-7) and (8-8), the resistance, R_{tube}, is then expressed as:

$$R_{tube} = \frac{\Delta P}{\dot{m}_{tube}} = 2 \times 10^9 \dot{m}_{tube} + 214329 + \frac{0.9082}{\dot{m}_{tube}} \qquad (8-9)$$

Simulation Model: Figure 8-8 is the model of the inspiratory line subsystem. P_H, the output from the humidification subsystem, and $P_{interface}$ from the patient interface subsystem, are the inputs into this system. The resistance of the inspiratory line is modeled using the Look-Up Table

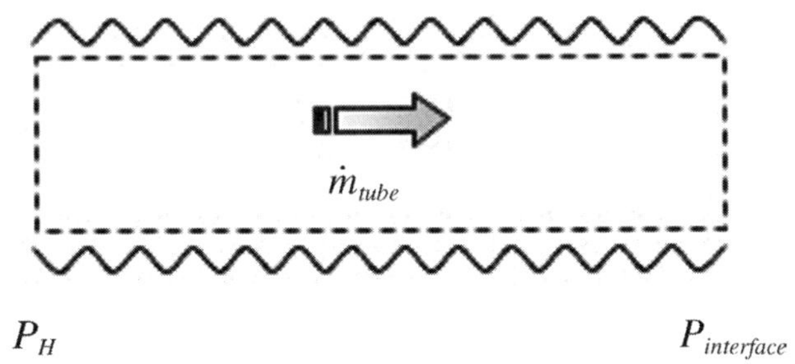

Figure 8-6. Modeling of the inspiratory line

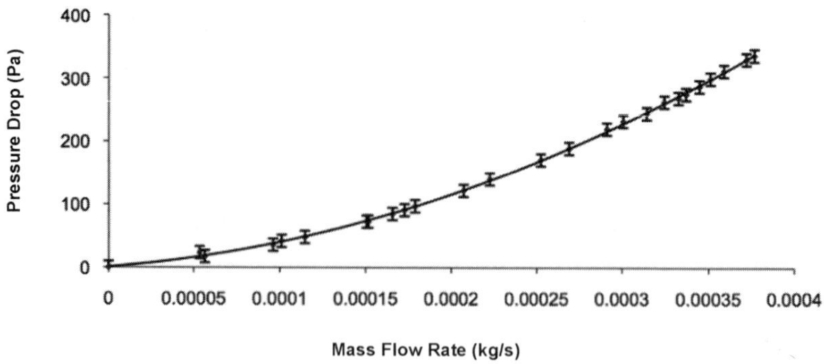

Figure 8-7. Inspiratory line pressure drop for various flow rates

block in Simulink™. This computes an approximation to some function y = f (x) given the data vectors x and y. For present purposes, y is R_{tube} and x is $\dot{m}_{tube}$. If the value of $\dot{m}_{tube}$ matches the block's input, the output, R_{tube}, is the corresponding element in the output vector.

8.2.3 Patient Interface

Assumptions and Simplifications: The patient interface serves to deliver the airflow, CPAP, and pressure oscillations to the patient. It is thus the hub of the various essential flows in the system. The non-linear resistance of the nasal prongs changes with the different nare diameters and materials needs to be determined experimentally. Since such data is unavailable, the present analysis is restricted to modeling the nasal tubing as a reservoir (even though the capacitance is small), as seen in Figure 8-9. The nasal prong resistance can be added to the system, if desired, and can be modeled in the manner outlined in Section 8.2.2.

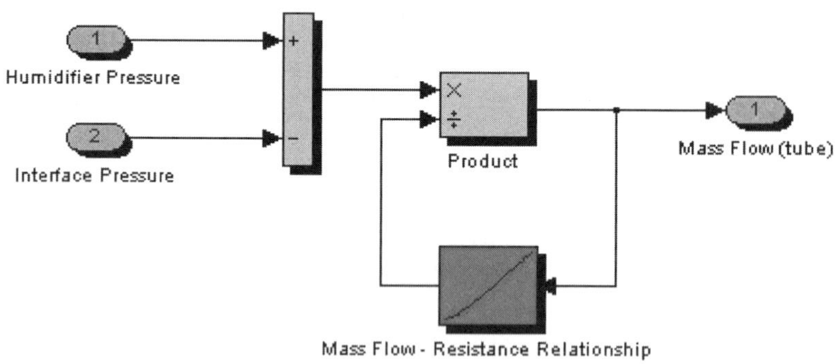

Figure 8-8. Inspiratory line subsystem

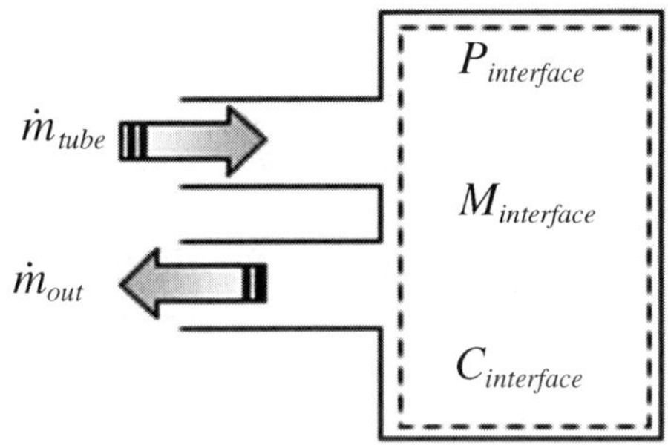

Figure 8-9. Modeling of the patient interface

Derivation: Similar to the model for the humidification chamber, the mass continuity equation for the patient interface is

$$\dot{m}_{tube} - \dot{m}_{out} = \frac{dM_{interface}}{dt} \tag{8 – 10}$$

where $\dot{m}_{out}$ is the air mass flow rate going out to the expiratory line; and $M_{interface}$ is the mass of air in the patient interface.

Using the equation of state, the mass of air in the interface is expressed as

$$P_{interface}V_{interface} = M_{interface}R_aT_{interface} \tag{8 – 11}$$

where

$$M_{interface} = C_{interface}P_{interface} \tag{8 – 12}$$

and

$$C_{interface} = \frac{V_{interface}}{R_aT_{interface}} \tag{8 – 13}$$

This renders the final model of the patient interface as:

$$\dot{m}_{tube} - \dot{m}_{out} = C_{interface}\frac{dP_{interface}}{dt} \tag{8 – 14}$$

Simulation Model: Figure 8-10 shows the model of the patient interface subsystem. The inputs are $\dot{m}_{tube}$ from the inspiratory line subsystem and $\dot{m}_{out}$ from the expiratory line subsystem. $P_{interface}$ is the output, which functions as the input for the inspiratory and expiratory line subsystems.

8.2.4 Expiratory Line

Assumptions and Simplifications: The expiratory line is commonly made of EVA copolymer and is smooth on the inside, but corrugated on the

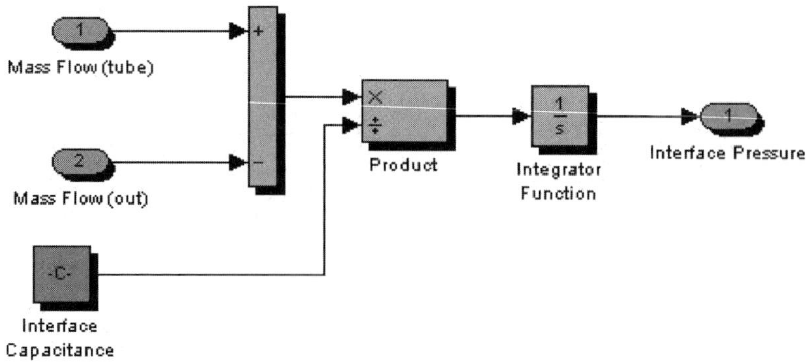

Figure 8-10. Patient interface subsystem

outside. Due to the presence of pressure oscillations in the expiratory line, the inertance of the fluid needs to be incorporated. Considering a control volume around the air in the expiratory line (Figure 8-11), the kinetic energy over the finite lump of fluid needs to be summed. Since we assume one-dimensional flow, all particles in the lump have the same velocity at any point in time and so the lump of fluid can be treated as if it were a rigid body of mass (m_{out}), such that:

$$m_{out} = \rho_{air} A_{tube} L \tag{8 – 15}$$

where ρ_{air} is the density of the air; A_{tube} is the cross-sectional area of the internal diameter; and L is the length of the tube.

Derivation: A pressure drop across the control volume will cause a fluid acceleration according to Newton's Second Law:

$$(P_{interface} - P_{CPAP} - \Delta P_{\exp}) A_{tube} = m_{out} a \tag{8 – 16}$$

where P_{CPAP} is the pressure generated at the CPAP generator; $\Delta P_{\exp}$ is the pressure drop in the tube; and a is the acceleration of the fluid mass.

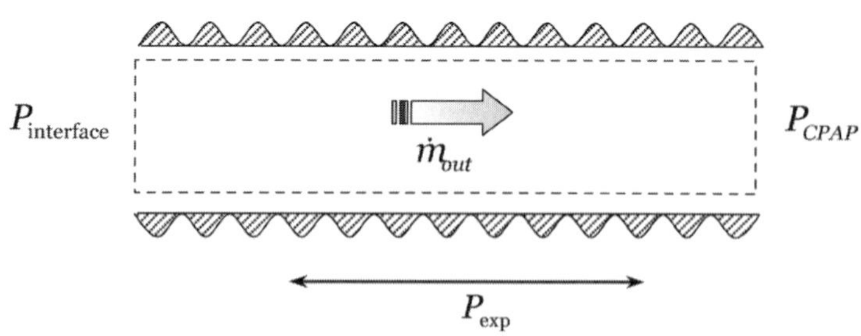

Figure 8-11. Modeling of the expiratory line

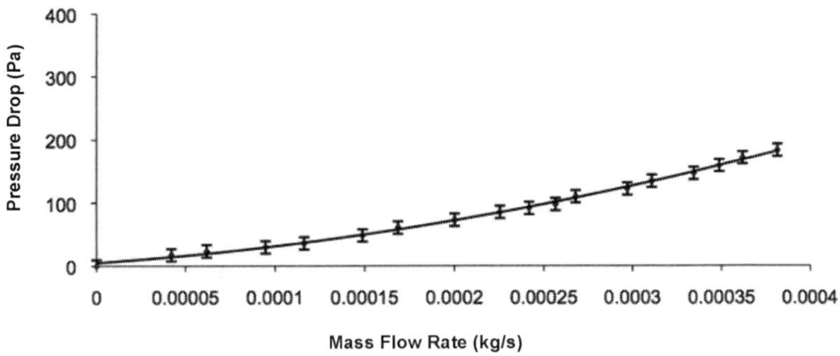

Figure 8-12. Expiratory limb pressure drop for various flow rates

Combining equations (8-15) and (8-16) renders the final form of the equation for the expiratory line as:

$$(P_{interface} - P_{CPAP} - \Delta P_{\exp})\frac{A_{tube}}{L} = \frac{d\dot{m}_{out}}{dt} \qquad (8-17)$$

ΔP_{exp} is also dependant on the air mass flow rate in the tube ($\dot{m}_{out}$). Again, a convenient method of determining this relationship is through empirical methods, as with the modeling of the inspiratory line. The static pressure drop across the expiratory line of the Bubble CPAP system was measured over a range of flow rates by Manilal [3]. This is shown in Figure 8-12 and expressed as the following empirical relationship:

$$\Delta P_{\exp} = 7\times 10^{8}\dot{m}_{out}^{2} + 191081\dot{m}_{out} + 4.9936 \qquad (8-18)$$

Simulation Model: Figure 8-13 shows the model of the expiratory line subsystem. $P_{interface}$ is modeled as an input to the subsystem along

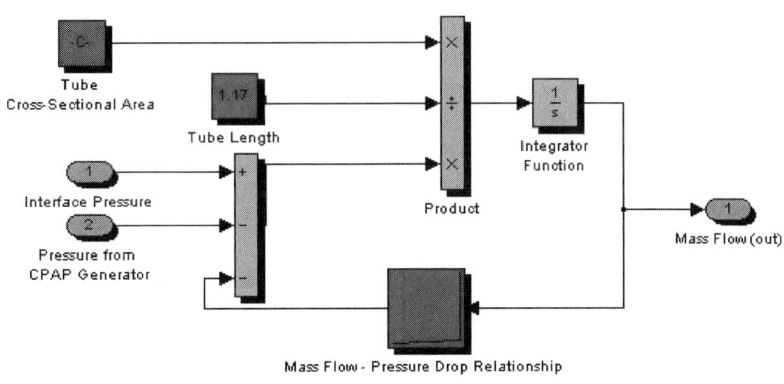

Figure 8-13. Expiratory tube subsystem

with P_{CPAP}. ΔP_{exp} is modeled using the Look-Up Table block with $\dot{m}_{out}$ as the input vector and ΔP_{exp} as the output vector. $\dot{m}_{out}$ is the output of the subsystem, which is fed back to the patient interface subsystem as an input.

8.2.5 The CPAP Generator

Assumptions and Simplifications: The CPAP generator needs to model the mean level of pressure and the pressure oscillations produced from such a system. The amplitude and frequency of the pressure oscillations in the Bubble CPAP system are dependent on the flow rate used. A relationship between the mass flow rate and frequency of pressure oscillations produced in the CPAP generator have not yet been established in the literature, and hence are difficult to quantify in terms of equations, so experimental data is required to use as realistic inputs into the model.

Simulation Model: Pressure readings taken at the distal end of the expiratory line (i.e., the end that connects to the CPAP probe) in a Bubble CPAP system under typical operating conditions (5c m H_2O of CPAP and 8 L/min of airflow rate) are shown in Figure 8-14 [2, 3] and used directly in the model as the input parameter P_{CPAP}.

8.2.6 Simplified Lung Model

Assumptions and Simplifications: A model of the lung is required to complete the system model such that interactions between patient and device can be assessed. Lumped parameter models of the lung of varying complexity have been previously developed in the literature and are dealt with in further detail in Chapter 9. Since the primary aim here is to illustrate methods of modeling using a systems dynamic approach, a simplified second-order model of the lung is used: It describes the elements of the respiratory system in terms of single equivalent inertial, viscous, and elastic components.

Derivation: A simplified lung model of the neonatal lung has been previously described as:

$$Q_{lung} = \frac{(P_{lung\ wall} + P_{interface})A^2}{m_{wall}D^2 + B_{wall}D + k_{wall}} \quad (8-19)$$

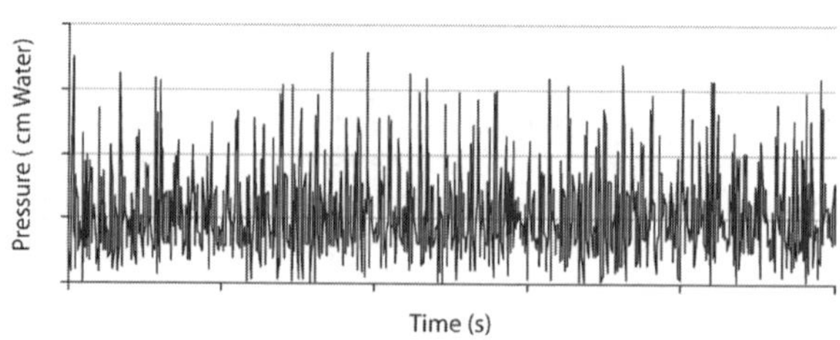

Figure 8-14. Pressure measurements for 10-mm probe at 8 l/min

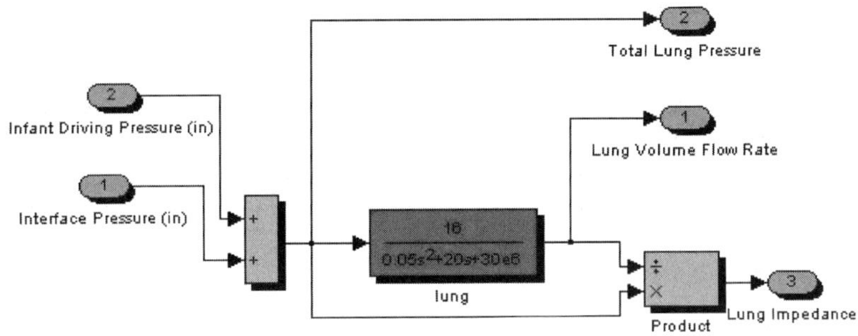

Figure 8-15. Lung subsystem

where Q_{lung} is the lung volume flow rate; $P_{lung\ wall}$ is the pressure responsible for the expansion and contraction of the lung wall; A is the surface area of the lung; m_{wall} is the lung mass; B_{wall} is the lung damping coefficient; K_{wall} is the lung stiffness; and D is the D operator $\left(\frac{d}{dt}\right)$.

Simulation Model: Figure 8-15 shows the model of the lung subsystem. $P_{lung\ wall}$ and $P_{interface}$ are inputs to the subsystem; and P_{total} (which is $P_{lung\ wall} + P_{interface}$), Q_{lung} and $Z_{effective}$ (an effective lung impedance) are outputs of the subsystem.

8.2.7 Complete System Simulation Model

Figure 8-16 shows the complete simulation model with all components of the Bubble CPAP System and the neonatal lung model. $P_{patient}$, $\dot{m}_{in}$, and P_{CPAP} are the time domain inputs to the system; P_{total}, Q_{lung}, and $Z_{effective}$, are outputs in the time domain.

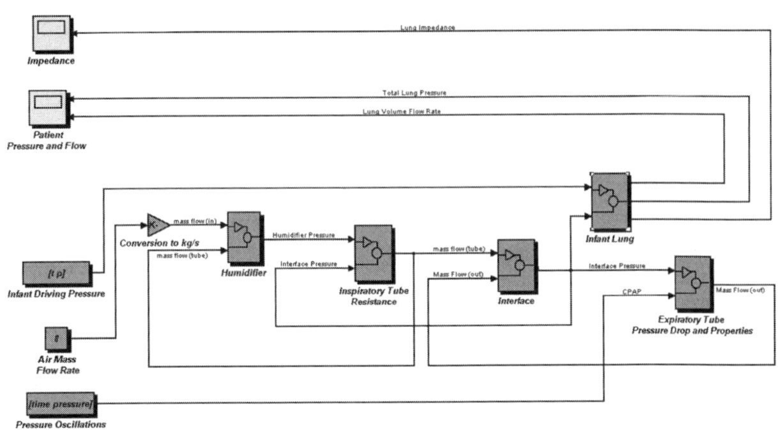

Figure 8-16. Complete simulation model

8.3 MODEL VALIDATION

Figure 8-18 shows the pressure waveform for 1 breath cycle at the patient interface produced by the model and a typical airway measurement from Lee et al. [4] of a neonate under normal typical conditions (5 cm H_2O of CPAP and 8 L/min of airflow rate). Both simulation and measurements

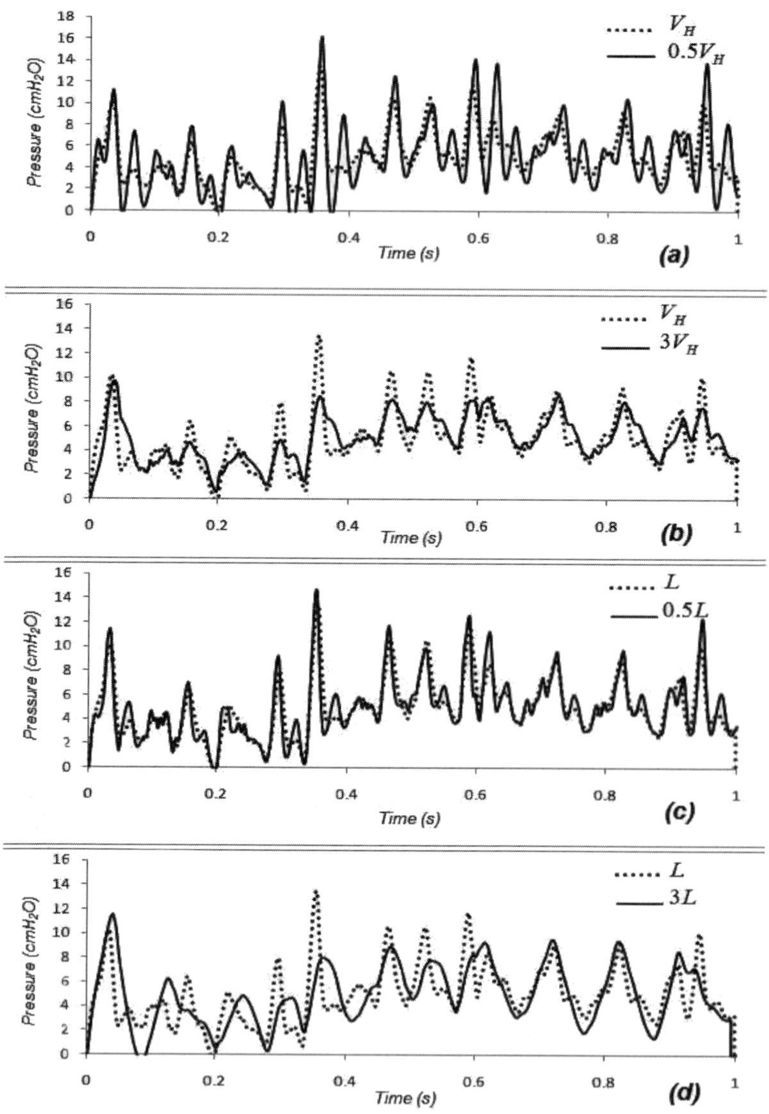

Figure 8-17. Effect of design parameters on pressure transmission

show pressure oscillation amplitudes within the same order of magnitude, and frequency analysis shows that strong frequencies lie between 15 and 30 Hz in the measurements and 15 and 45 Hz in the simulation.

For the present purposes, such a qualitative comparison may be adequate; however, depending on the purposes of simulation studies and the type of medical device being modeled, tighter tolerances may be set by the investigator.

8.4 MODEL UTILITY

This section presents a few examples of how the model can be used in practice as a design tool, to reduce the time and effort involved in the "trial and error" process of laboratory testing that is common with respiratory devices.

8.4.1 Effect of Design Parameters on Pressure Transmission

This section illustrates how the model can be used to detect the sensitivity of the system operation to changing design parameters. The humidifier volume (L) and expiratory line tube length (V_H) are used as examples. Separate simulations are performed where the humidifier volume and tube length are adjusted to new values of 0.5 and 3 times the original values (i.e. 0.5 V_H, 3 V_H, 0.5 L and 3 L). Figure 8-17 compares the interface pressure under normal operating conditions with pressures produced by changing the aforementioned parameters. It can be seen that the pressure oscillation amplitudes and frequencies are damped with an increasing humidifier volume and expiratory tube length. Such simulations can give an idea of the magnitude of change to be expected in system outputs based on the changes to design features, and help to better design and reduce the number of laboratory tests in engineering practice.

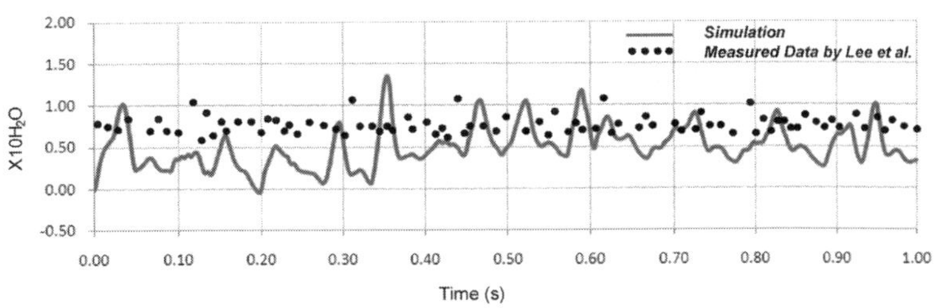

Figure 8-18. Comparison of waveform produced at patient interface by simulation and measurements from Lee et al. [4]

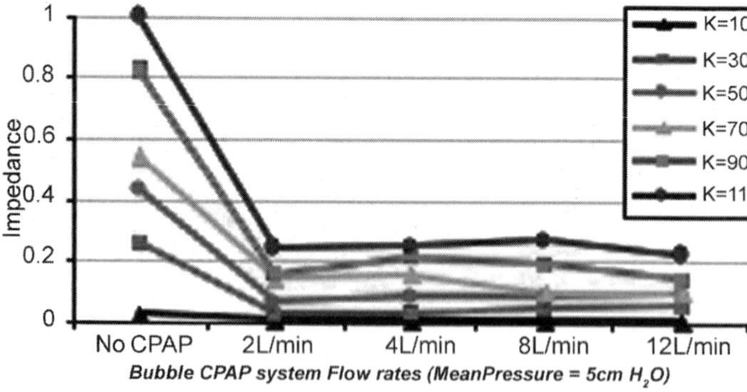

Figure 8-19. Lung performance at different bubble CPAP system settings

8.4.2 Interaction with Neonatal Lung

Manilal-Reddy and Al-Jumaily [2] used the model to investigate neonatal lung performance when exposed to Bubble CPAP by considering the normalized impedance at the patient interface. The normalized impedance versus Bubble CPAP flow rate for different patient – Bubble CPAP configurations is shown in Figure 8-19.

Healthy lungs were assumed to have an overall stiffness in the range of $k_{wall} = 10 - 60$ MPa and the lung is considered unhealthy if it has values above that range. The overall findings were that for unhealthy lungs, Bubble CPAP settings between 8 and 12 L/min appeared most beneficial to lung performance, mainly due to the presence of strong contributions of pressure oscillation frequencies at 30 and 60 Hz. The differences in effective impedance values before applying pressure oscillations are vast across all k_{wall} values. However, these differences in lung performance become very small after pressure oscillations are applied.

The neonatal lung, however, is much more complex than the one described in the simple one-compartmental model here, where differences in maturity are reflected in airway resistance, compliance, lung capacity, lung stiffness, and lung mass properties. This limits the use of the model to make more accurate and in-depth simulation studies. A more comprehensive model of the neonatal airway is presented in the next chapter, which will extend the use of the modeling techniques used here.

8.5 CLOSURE

This chapter follows a step-by-step approach to modeling the different aspects of a Bubble CPAP device. Comparisons of the model with actual measurements show that the model is able to predict the realistic operation of the device. An example of how the model can be used to modify design features is given at the end of the chapter.

REFERENCES

[1] Aly, H.Z., Nasal Prongs Continuous Positive Airway Pressure: A Simple Yet Powerful Tool. *Pediatrics*, 2001. **108**(3): p. 759–761.

[2] Manilal-Reddy, P.I. and A.M. Al-Jumaily, Understanding the use of continuous oscillating positive airway pressure (bubble CPAP) to treat neonatal respiratory disease: An engineering approach. *Journal of Medical Engineering & Technology*, 2009. **33**(3): p. 214–22.

[3] Manilal, P., The Effect of Pressure Oscillations on Neonatal Breathing, Master of Engineering Thesis, in Diagnostics and Control Research Centre. 2004, Auckland University of Technology: Auckland. p. 134.

[4] Lee, K.S., Dunn, M.S., Fenwick, M., Shennan, A.T., A comparison of underwater bubble continuous positive airway pressure with ventilator-derived continuous positive airway pressure in premature neonates ready for extubation. *Biology of the Neonate*, 1998. **73**(69): p. 69–75.

Chapter 9

MODELING DEVICE INTERACTION WITH THE NEONATAL LUNG

This chapter provides an introduction to the structure, function, and mechanics of the respiratory system, before proceeding to discuss existing models in the literature that have been developed to answer a variety of questions on respiratory performance. The procedure of developing a validated lumped parameter mathematical model of a non-linear biological system such as the lung is described, and its implementation in the Simulink™ environment is also elaborated on. This is followed by an explanation of how such a model can be integrated with a model of a respiratory device (such as the Bubble CPAP system developed in Chapter 8) to determine the effect of device operation on respiratory performance. In particular, the model is used to study the transmission of pressure oscillations in combination with Continuous Positive Airway Pressure (CPAP) through the neonatal tracheobronchial tree.

9.1 RESPIRATORY SYSTEM STRUCTURE AND FUNCTION

The primary function of the respiratory system is to supply the blood with oxygen and to enable carbon dioxide to move out. It is made up of a gas exchange organ (the lungs) and a respiratory pump (the chest wall and respiratory muscles). The organs and process of respiration are explained in this section [1-3].

9.1.1 Anatomy

The respiratory system consists of several organs that include the nasal cavity, throat (pharynx), voice box (larynx), windpipe (trachea), bronchi,

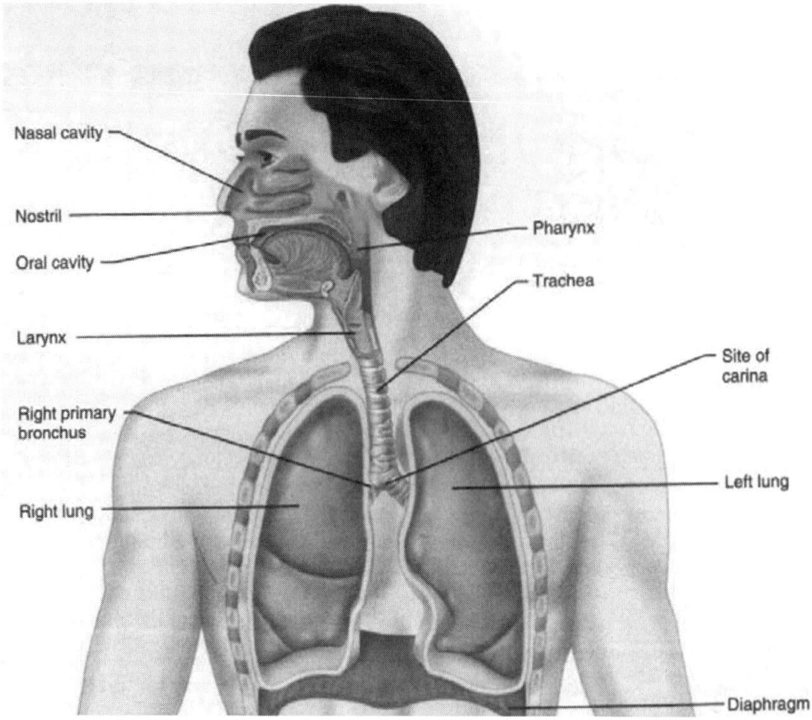

Figure 9-1. Respiratory system organs [Reproduced with permission from Marieb et al. [3]]

lungs, and respiratory muscles. This is illustrated in Figure 9-1. The nostrils and proceeding nasal cavity herald the beginning of the human respiratory tract. Their primary functions are to filter out mechanical aerial contaminants and to warm and humidify the inhaled air. The intervening pharynx acts primarily as a conduit between the aforementioned passages and the trachea. The trachea itself is a musculo-cartilaginous tube, which further moistens the inflowing air and additionally filters smaller diameter particles.

The trachea in turn branches at the carina (Figure 9-1) into the primary conducting airways supplying each lung, i.e., the right and left primary bronchi. Hereafter, each bronchus divides again, forming secondary, tertiary, and smaller bronchi (Figure 9-2) such that they become smaller and more numerous as they penetrate deeper into the lungs, forming lobar, then segmental bronchi. Figure 9-2 also shows the five lobes of the lungs (three in the right lung and two in the left lung).

The division of the bronchi continues down to the terminal bronchioles (the smallest airways without alveoli). The airways from the trachea to the terminal bronchioles are called the conducting airways. Their function is to lead the inspired air from the exterior to the gas exchange region

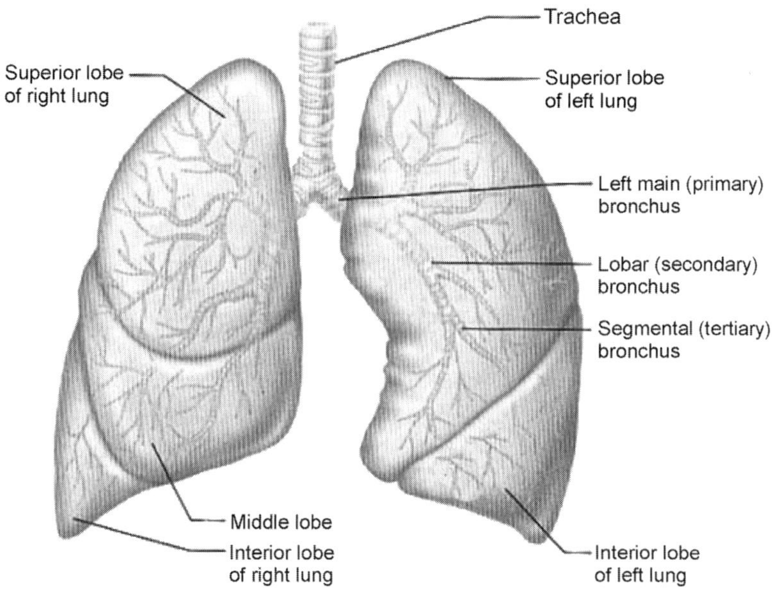

Figure 9-2. Branching of conducting airways in the lung [Reproduced with permission from Marieb et al. [3]]

or respiratory zone of the lung (shown in Figure 9-3). The respiratory zone is made up of respiratory bronchioles (which have occasional alveoli budding from their walls), alveolar ducts, and alveoli. There are about 300 million alveoli in the human lung, each about 1/3 mm diameter.

The distance from the terminal bronchiole to the most distal alveolus is only a few millimeters but the respiratory zone constitutes most of the lung. The alveoli are surrounded by pulmonary capillaries, which form

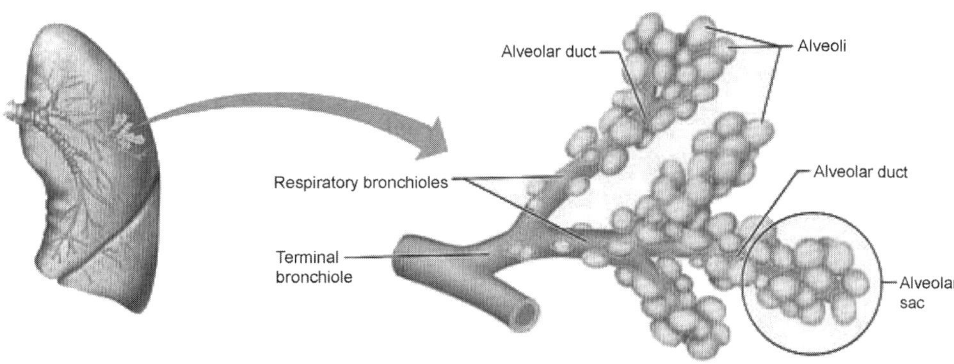

Figure 9-3. Respiratory zone of the lung [Reproduced with permission from Marieb et al. [3]]

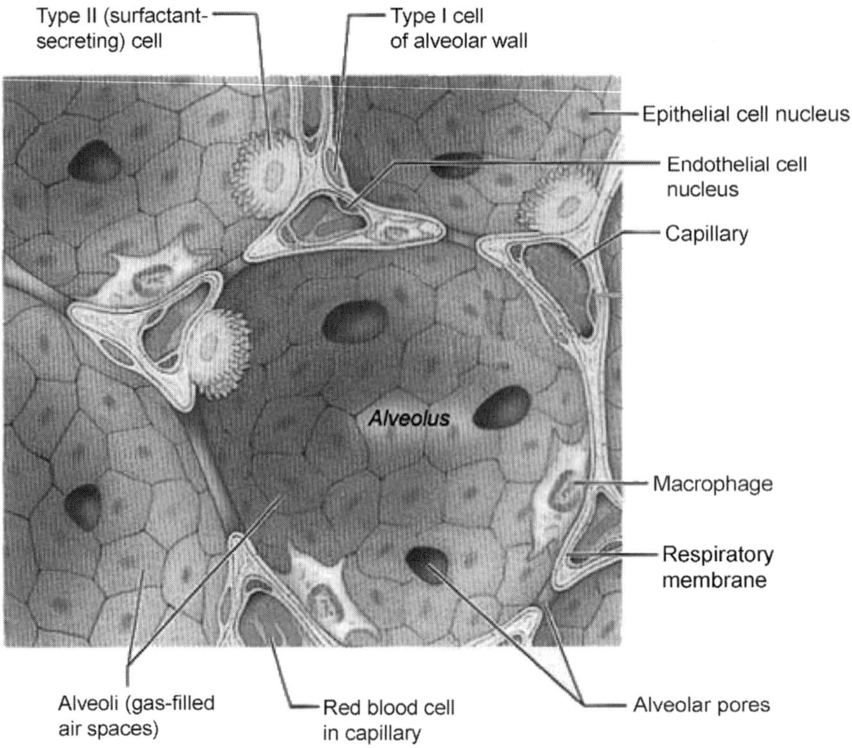

Figure 9-4. Cells in the alveoli [Reproduced with permission from Marieb et al. [3]]

a dense network in the walls of the alveoli, such that the capillaries form an almost continuous sheet of blood on the alveolar wall surface (which is about 70 to 85 m^2 in adult humans). The barrier between the air and the blood is only about 0.5 μm apart such that oxygen and carbon dioxide can diffuse through the barrier with ease.

Four generations of respiratory bronchioles develop before birth and several million alveoli form in the last few weeks of birth, underscoring the importance of the last few weeks of gestation [4].

Premature infants born before or during this important stage of alveolarization are subjected to mechanical ventilation before the development of alveoli. This could disrupt the normal process of lung development and lead to bronchopulmonary dysplasia (BPD) [1, 3-5]. Two types of epithelial cells line the alveoli (as seen in Figure 9-4). Type I cells are the primary lining cells. Type II cells are thicker and secrete surfactant. The alveoli also contain macrophages, which clean off inhaled dust particles and microorganisms. Figure 9-4 also shows the pulmonary capillaries and red blood cells (erythrocytes).

9.1.2 Inspiration, Expiration, and the Respiratory Muscles

The inspiration and expiration processes during quiet breathing are illustrated in Figure 9-5 and Figure 9-6, respectively, and explained as follows [1, 3, 5]. Inspiration is an active process. The most important muscle of inspiration is the diaphragm, which accounts for 75% of the change in intrathoracic volume. It is a thin, dome-shaped sheet of muscle that is attached at the bottom of the thoracic cage.

It moves downward like a piston when it contracts and the vertical dimension of the chest cavity is increased (Figure 9-5(a)). The external intercostals muscles run obliquely forward and downward, connecting the ribs. When they contract, they pull the ribs upward and forward (in a "bucket-handle" motion) such that the sternum is also pushed outward. The scalene muscles also elevate the first two ribs. There is little activity by the scalene muscles during quiet breathing but they may contract vigorously during exercise.

The increase in intrathoracic volume by the contraction of all the respiratory muscles causes a decrease in pressure in the lung according to the ideal gas law, since the volume increases due to temperature changes are small (Figure 9-5(b)). This causes air to rush into the lung from the atmosphere since fluid flows down along a pressure gradient. As a result, the pressure within the lung (intrapulmonary pressure) decreases to

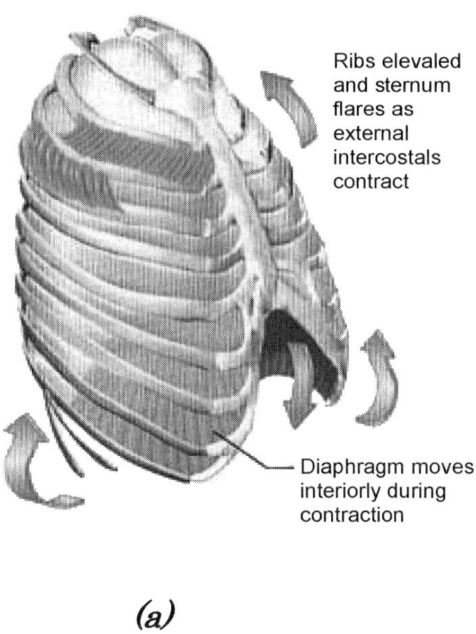

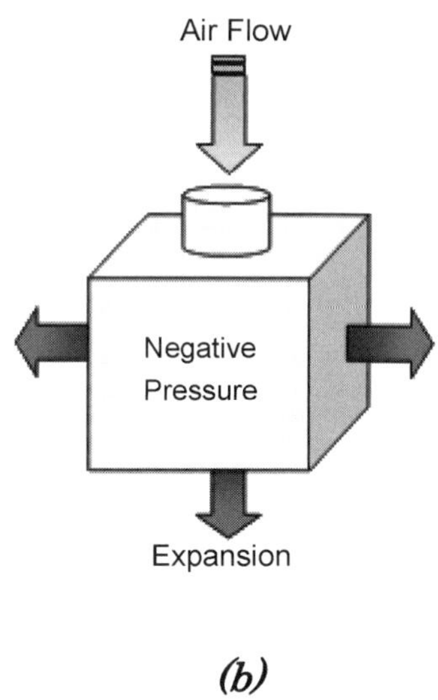

Figure 9-5. Inspiration process during quiet breathing: (a) thorax during inspiration [Reproduced with permission from Marieb et al; [3]]; (b) schematic of inspiration

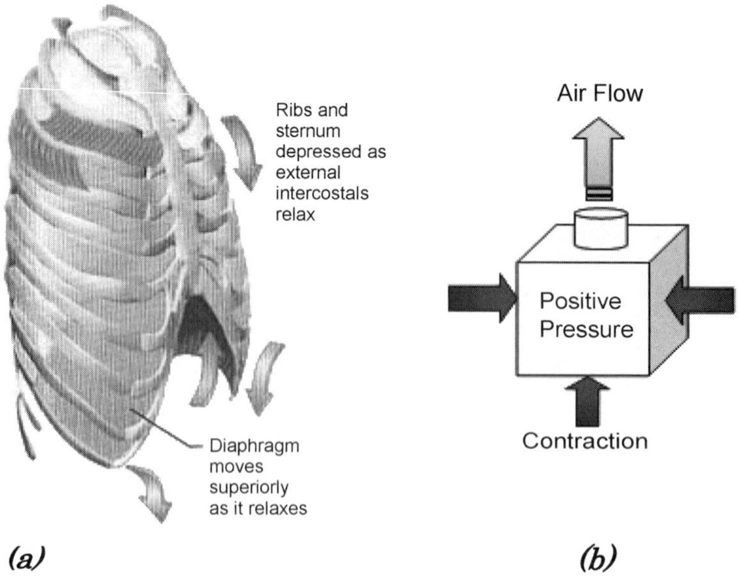

Figure 9-6. Expiration process during quiet breathing: (a) thorax during expiration [Reproduced with permission from Marieb et al. [3]]; (b) schematic of expiration

negative values during inspiration. The inspiration process ends when the intrapulmonary pressure and the atmospheric pressure become equal.

Expiration is a passive process in that it depends on the elasticity of the lungs and the chest wall. As the diaphragm and other inspiratory muscles relax, the lungs and chest wall recoil to their resting position (Figure 9-6(a)). Thus the lung volume is decreased and the intrapulmonary pressure increases to positive values during expiration. The pressure gradient now forces air out of the lungs (Figure 9-6(b)). During exercise, however, expiration becomes active.

The internal intercostals muscles contract, pulling the rib cage downward and thereby decreasing the thoracic volume. Muscles in the abdomen also contract, raising the intra-abdominal pressure, thus pushing the diaphragm upward.

The lungs and the chest wall are elastic structures that are connected by a common pleural cavity and pleurae, as seen in Figure 9-7. The pleura is a membrane that folds back on itself to create a double-layered membrane. The parietal pleura (outer pleura) is attached to the chest wall and the visceral pleura (inner pleura) is attached to the lung surface. The thin space between the pleurae (the pleural cavity) is filled with a lubricating fluid called the pleural fluid. The pleural fluid allows the lung to slide easily on the chest wall and prevent pleural separation due to the surface tension of the pleural fluid. This is akin to two moist pieces of glass that

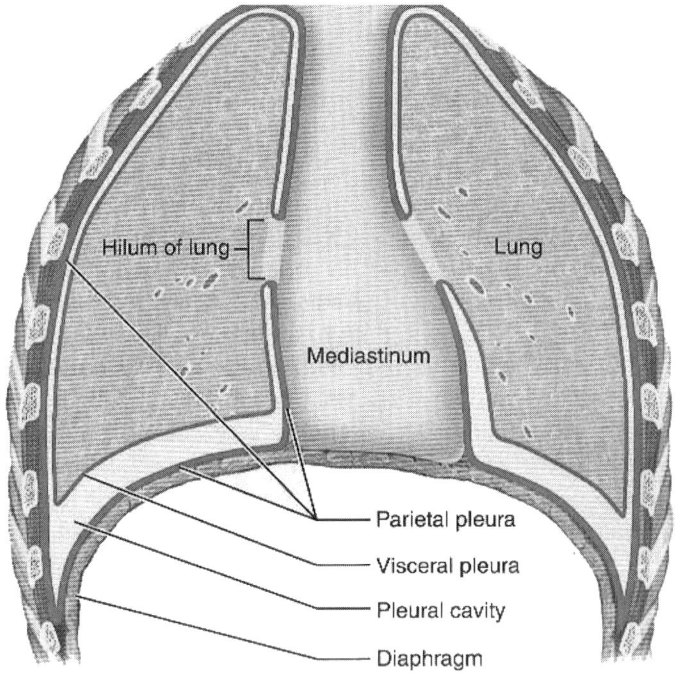

Figure 9-7. The pleural cavity [Reproduced with permission from Marieb et al. [3]]

can slide on each other but resist being separated. Thus, the pressure in the pleural cavity (the intrapleural pressure) is subatmospheric. The tendency for the chest wall to recoil at the end of quiet expiration is balanced by the tendency for the lung to recoil away from the chest wall. If the chest wall is opened, the lungs collapse and if the lungs lose their elastic recoil, the chest expands and becomes barrel shaped.

9.1.3 Respiratory Volumes and Capacities

The respiratory or lung volumes and the names applied to combinations of them (the respiratory capacities) are shown in Figure 9-8 [4, 5]. During quiet breathing, the amount of air that moves into the lungs with normal inspiration (or the amount that moves out during expiration) is called the tidal volume (TV). The amount of air that can be forcibly inspired beyond the tidal volume is the inspiratory reserve volume (IRV). The volume of air that can be forcibly exhaled after quiet expiration is the expiratory reserve volume (ERV). The air left in the lungs after a forced expiration is the residual volume (RV), which helps to keep the airways open and hence prevent lung collapse. The volume of the conducting zone of the

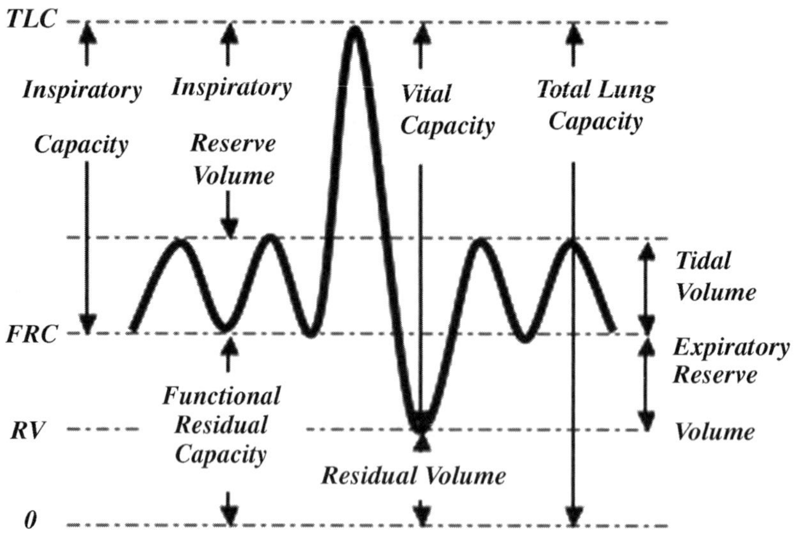

Figure 9-8. Respiratory volumes and capacities

lungs is called the respiratory dead space, since there is no diffusion of respiratory gases into and out of the blood in this section of the lung. Respiratory capacities always incorporate two or more lung volumes.

The inspiratory capacity (IC) is the sum of the TV and the IRV and is the amount of air that can be inspired after a quiet expiration. The amount of air that remains in the lungs after a quiet expiration is the functional residual capacity (FRC). This combines the RV and the ERV. The vital capacity (VC) is the sum of the TV, ERV, and IRV, which is effectively the total amount of exchangeable air. The sum of all the lung volumes is known as the total lung capacity (TLC).

9.2 RESPIRATORY MECHANICS

This section introduces the mechanical aspects of airflow in the respiratory system. The parameters introduced are commonly used parameters in clinical practice and experimentation, to assess respiratory mechanics and performance. They deal with the forces that move the lung and chest wall and the resisting forces that they have to overcome.

9.2.1 Airway Resistance

Airway resistance is the major source of non-elastic impediment encountered in the lung. It can be measured at the airway opening as the total resistance encountered in all the airway branches combined. In the lung, a pressure difference exists between the atmosphere and the alveoli where the airways are a series of branching tubes in between. Each airway can be considered as a tube where a pressure difference (ΔP_{airway}) exists between the ends, which is a function of the rate and the pattern of flow (Q). In laminar flow, ΔP_{airway} is proportional to Q and a constant K such that:

$$\Delta P_{airway} = KQ \qquad (9-1)$$

However, in turbulent flow, ΔP_{airway} is not proportional to Q, but to its square. In a complex system of branching tubes such as the bronchial tree, with its various bifurcation angles, surface roughness, and diameters, the application of a simple expression for ΔP_{airway} is difficult. Laminar flow is most likely to occur in the terminal bronchioles and fully developed turbulent flow is most likely to occur in the trachea. However, for most of the bronchial tree, the flow is most likely to be transitional.

9.2.2 Compliance

The compliance is the ratio of the change in pressure (ΔP) and the change in volume (ΔV) and reflects the elastic properties of the respiratory system. The lung compliance (C_L) is expressed as

$$C_L = \frac{\Delta V}{\Delta P} = \frac{1}{E_L} \qquad (9-2)$$

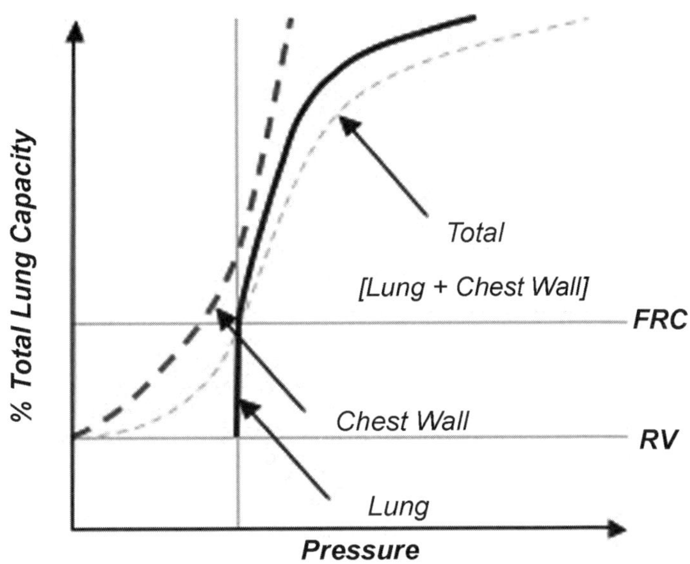

Figure 9-9. Neonatal lung and chest wall compliance

where the elastance of the lung (E_L) is the reciprocal of the lung compliance (C_L). Static lung compliance measurements can be made by measuring the transpulmonary pressure (which is the pressure difference between the alveolar and pleural pressure), before and after inflation with a known volume. This is measured at the mouth and esophagus. The chest wall compliance (C_{CW}) can be measured in a similar manner by recording the difference between pleural and atmospheric pressures. A pressure-volume curve can be made by recording the pressures at several different volumes. Figure 9-9 shows typical lung and chest wall expansion curves for a neonatal lung. The sum of the two is the total compliance (C_T). It is apparent that the compliance is not linear across the entire range of expansion, with the compliance getting smaller at higher expanding pressures, as seen by the flatter slope of the curves at higher pressures. Compliance is a useful measure of diseased states. It is reduced in conditions of pulmonary fibrosis, alveolar edema, and atelectasis, which prevent the inflation of the lung. Compliance increases in pulmonary emphysema and in the aging lung, where the elastic properties of the tissue alter.

9.2.3 Impedance

The impedance of the respiratory system (Z_L) is an expression of the overall impediment to flow in the respiratory system. It is the result of a combination of the resistive, elastic, and inertive elements and is given by

$$Z_L = \left|\frac{P}{Q}\right| \qquad (9-3)$$

where P is the instantaneous pressure at the airway opening.

9.2.4 Alveolar Surface Tension

Alveolar surface tension is the force acting across an imaginary line (1 cm in length) on the liquid lining of surfactant, and hence has the SI unit of N/m but is commonly expressed in the literature as "dynes/cm." It is an important factor that affects the pressure-volume relationship of the lung. This can be measured by inflating excised lungs with saline at various volumes, to abolish the air-liquid interface in the alveoli, thereby reducing the surface tension to almost zero. A typical resulting pressure-volume curve, such as that seen in Figure 9-10 [1, 5], is one that measures only the tissue elasticity, whereas similar measurements done with air, measure the effects of both tissue elasticity and surface tension. Figure 9-10 shows that saline-filled lungs have a higher compliance and less hysteresis than air-filled lungs, indicating that surface tension contributes to a large part of the static recoil force of the lung.

The surface tension-reducing mechanism of surfactant can be better understood by looking at the intermolecular forces between the surfactant molecules. Pulmonary surfactant is made up of 90% phospholipids and

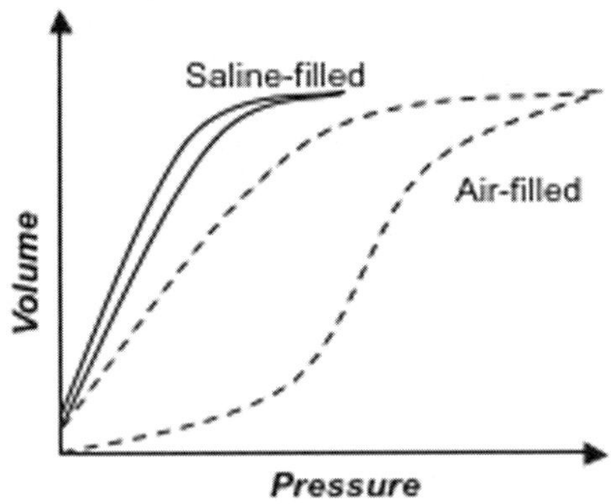

Figure 9-10. Pressure-volume curves of air-filled and saline-filled lungs

10% proteins. Phospholipid is the primary surface-tension lowering component of pulmonary surfactant and makes up most of its mass. The proteins enhance the surface tension lowering ability of the surfactant. The surfactant-associated proteins are SP-A, SP-B, SP-C, and SP-D. Figure 9-11 shows the composition of mammalian surfactant. Although there is some variation in surfactant across species, the compositions given are representative, since composition in mammals in general is considered to be similar.

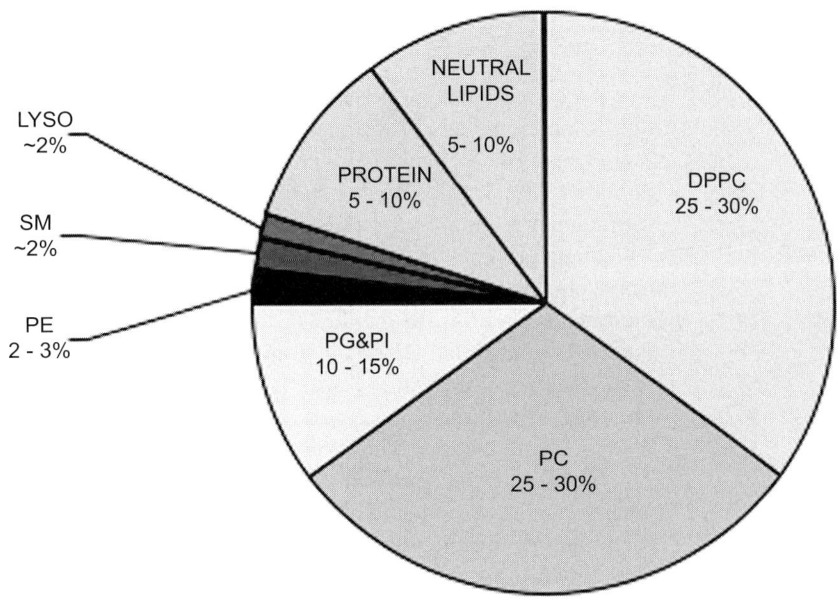

Figure 9-11. Mammalian surfactant composition

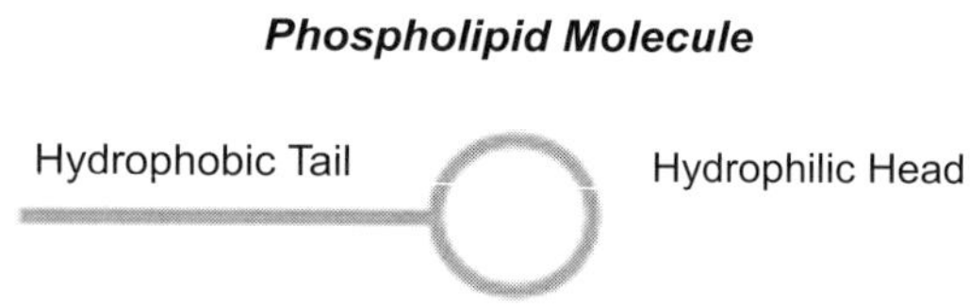

Figure 9-12. Phospholipid molecule

Phospholipid content can be divided in 25% to 30% dipalmitoyl-phospatidylcholine (DPPC), 25% to 30% unsaturated phospatidylcholine (PC), 10% to 15% phosphatidylglycerol (PG), plus phosphatidylinositol (PI), 5% to 10% neutral lipids, 5% to 10% proteins, and about 2% each of sphingomyelin (SM) and lyso-bis-phosphatic acid (LYSO).

Phospholipids are mainly responsible for giving the surfactant its surface tension-reducing capacity and this is discussed in greater detail as follows: Phospholipid molecules contain a hydrophobic tail and a hydrophilic head (Figure 9-12) and exist as aggregates because they are insoluble in the aqueous mixture that lines the alveoli.

At the air-liquid interface of the alveoli, water molecules are attracted to each other and to molecules in the bulk liquid, thereby creating a contractive force known as surface tension. The surface tension acts to reduce the surface area of the air-liquid interface to create a stable position at minimal surface area. Surface tension has a value of 0.7 mN/cm for water at 37°C (more commonly expressed as 70 dynes/cm). This resists expansion of the alveoli in the lung in diseased states where there is no surfactant.

To increase the surface area sufficiently for adequate ventilation requires large amounts of distending pressure to be generated, and hence, more work. This explains why a premature infant, who is unable to produce pulmonary surfactant, is faced with the further difficulty of having to perform more muscle work to counter the tendency of the alveoli to collapse.

In the presence of surfactant in a healthy lung, the hydrophilic heads of the phospholipids interact with the water molecules and the hydrophobic tails extend toward the air (as seen in Figure 9-13). This displaces the water molecules at the air-liquid interface (which are attracted to each other by electrostatic forces known as Van de Waals forces), thus reducing the surface tension to equilibrium values of approximately 25 dynes/cm [4, 6].

Surface tension forces in the alveoli can be described by the static Young-Laplace equation [5-7], most commonly applied to a small spherical air bubble in a surfactant suspension that is pulsated at regular frequencies, between a fixed minimum and maximum radius [equation (9-4)].

$$\Delta P = \frac{2\gamma}{r} \tag{9-4}$$

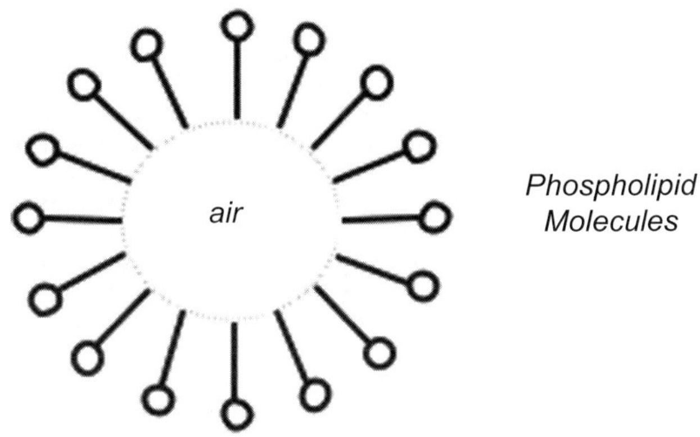

Figure 9-13. Phospholipid molecules at the air-liquid interface

Here ΔP is the pressure drop across the air-liquid interface that is needed to stabilize the system; r is the radius of the bubble; and γ is the surface tension.

In the absence of surfactant, the surface tension increases and equation (9-4) illustrates that more distending pressure is required to stop the alveoli from collapsing. If the radius of the alveolus is small, a larger distending pressure is necessary to keep it open. In a premature infant whose alveoli are deficient in surfactant and naturally smaller in radius than those of normal infants, surfactant therapies and ventilation are required to expand the alveoli to prevent collapse at the end of expiration. Equation (9-4) ignores the dynamic effects of surface dilational viscosity, κ, which affects the interfacial pressure drop when the bubble changes dynamically. A complete description of the interfacial behavior is given by equation (9-5), which is a function of radius, r; surface tension, γ; and surface dilational viscosity, κ [8]:

$$\Delta P = \frac{2\gamma}{r} + \frac{4\kappa\dot{r}}{r^2} \qquad (9-5)$$

These effects, if ignored during experiments, can result in significant errors; however, for the purposes of a basic explanation, the Young-Laplace equation suffices.

9.2.5 Work of Breath

Generally, the Work of Breath (WOB) refers to the mechanical work performed by the respiratory muscles against the lung and chest wall during respiration [1, 5]. It is most convenient to measure work as the product of pressure and volume change, which has the same units as work (Nm).

The WOB can be calculated from a relaxation pressure curve, such as that shown in Figure 9-9. The WOB is complex and difficult to measure without sophisticated analysis to quantify the movement and distortion of the chest wall [5, 9].

However, in many cases, measuring the work performed against an external load may provide sufficient information for the purposes of respiratory performance [9]. The work measured at the mouth or airway opening estimates the work performed by all the respiratory muscles. Alternatively, it can be measured using the transpulmonary pressure for measurement of the chest wall and its muscles against the lung and airways. The work of breath can be expressed as the work done per breath, work per minute, or work per liter [10].

9.3 MODELING RESPIRATORY SYSTEM DYNAMICS

This is an application of the "Talkative Models" approach introduced in Chapter 1. To model the lung, a variety of models are available in the literature, including poroelastic, computational fluid dynamics (CFD), morphometric, and mechanical models. A search of the literature reveals that the approach and complexity of modeling the respiratory system depends on the research question. The effects of gas mixing, efferent activity, and ventilation-perfusion effects are not studied in this work. Models that incorporate geometric, physical, mechanical, and flow characteristics are considered, so a review on the morphometric and mechanical models found in the literature is discussed in this section.

9.3.1 Morphometric Models

Morphometric models represent the branching structure of the airways along with other data, such as the dimensions and branching angles as well as cross-sectional areas and volumes of alveoli. Weibel [11] developed a symmetric model of the human adult lung that incorporated 23 generations of symmetrically dividing tubes and 300 million alveoli. The Weibel model is widely used in analytical and numerical prediction because of its convenient symmetric structure [6]. However, the airway branching in the real lung does not end abruptly at generation 23, so Hansen and Ampaya [12] refined the Weibel model by performing detailed analyses of the alveolar regions, concluding that the lung has 27 generations of airways. Also, the system developed by Weibel, with the doubling of the airways at each generation, was replaced by a system where the number of airways was increased at each generation up to generation 24, then decreased until generation 27. Hansen and Ampaya distinguished six different types of alveoli and concluded that there were in fact 450 million alveoli in the lung.

Horsfield et al. [13] developed a more realistic model where the branching structure of the airways is asymmetric, but this pattern of asymmetry is constant. In reality, the terminal bronchioles require a different pattern of asymmetry, so for more sophisticated computational analyses, computer models developed from computer tomography (CT) scans show more promise [14]. For the current purposes, however, the interest in airway branching structure is focused on the first few generations and so the Weibel and Horsfield models are adequate.

9.3.2 Mechanical Models

Computer models that use lumped parameters to describe lung mechanics are often used to investigate the effects of lung development and diseases on respiratory measurements. Such models can also be used to determine the interaction of the respiratory system with respiratory support equipment and ventilation techniques.

The simplest model to describe lung mechanics is a single compartment model (Figure 9-14(a)), consisting of a single compliance, *C*, and

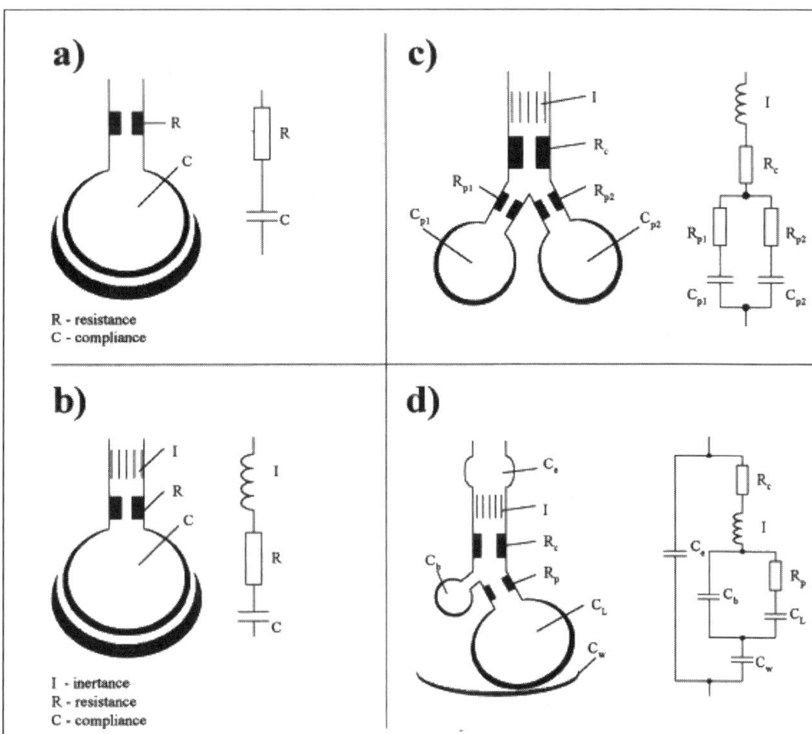

Figure 9-14. Lung models to model respiratory system mechanics [16]

a single resistance, R (the RC model) [15]. This model is suitable for simple tidal breathing predictions but is inadequate for higher frequency analysis due to the lack of inertance, I. Adding inertance to the model (the RIC model in Figure 9-14(b)) means that it is useful in the study of simple maturation studies due to the small number of required model parameters [16].

Mead [17] suggested a model with seven parameters (Figure 9-14(d)), namely inertance (I), central and peripheral resistances (R_c and R_p), and lung, chest wall, bronchial, and extrathoracic compliances (C_l, C_w, C_b, and C_e). Although it considers these further properties and is able to simulate the influences of mask leaks and compliance on the respiratory system, as well as the effects of bronchiole obstruction, it still remains an extended version of a single compartment model and cannot simulate uneven ventilation.

Viscoelastic models that separate airway and tissue properties into separate regions are also available in the literature. Athanasiades et al. [18] used a viscoelastic model (shown in Figure 9-15) to calculate the WOB in normal adults.

R_u, R_c, R_s, and R_{ve} are the upper airways, collapsible airways, small airways, and viscoelastic element resistances. C_c, C_l, C_{ve}, and C_{cw} are the collapsible airways, lung tissue, viscoelastic element, and chest wall compliances. P_{mus} and P_{atm} are the pressure due to muscle activity and the atmosphere. Liu et al. [19] used the same type of model, but added a pulmonary circulation model (to describe gas exchange at the alveolar-capillary membrane) that could accurately predict the expired gas concentrations. These models, however, do not include the inertance, which make them inadequate for simulations that involve frequencies much higher than breathing frequencies; like the Mead model [17], they are single compartment models that limits their use in ventilation distribution studies.

Tomlinson et al. [20] also uses a single compartment model of an adult lung to simulate pressure, flow, and volume. However, unlike Mead [17] and Athanasiades [18], the Tomlinson model includes flow-dependant resistance in the upper airways, as well as lung and chest wall viscoelasticity and inertance. More experimental data is still required to correlate with the model; however, it does show promise for use in dynamic studies.

A two-compartment model (Figure 9-14(c)) as proposed by Schmidt [16] and Crooke and Head [21] is well suited to investigations of uneven ventilation. The values of C, I, and R can be adjusted to reflect different pathologies. These models can predict tidal volumes, flows, and pressures in each compartment that could be of interest to clinicians. The models, however, do not include airway and chest wall compliance. These types of models, although improvements on the single compartment model, do not consider flow dependant resistance, which is important in describing the upper airways [22].

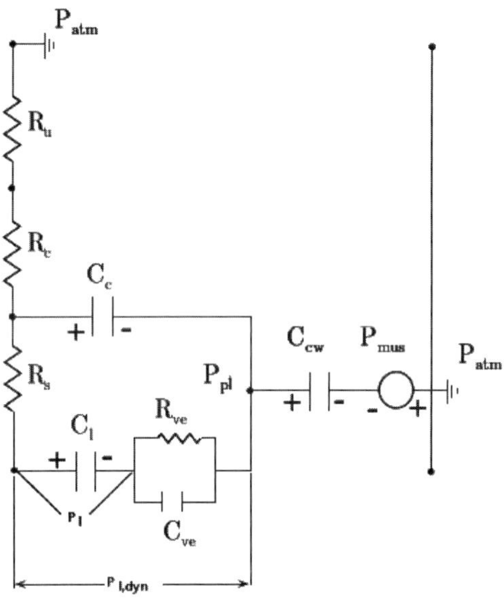

Figure 9-15. Viscoelastic model as used by athanasiades et al. [18]

A model by Polak and Lutchen [23] uses an asymmetric Horsfield bronchial tree that leads to several independent alveolar compartments. Viscoelastic properties of the lobes and the inertia of airway walls are neglected. Also, it is assumed that mechanical properties do not vary between compartments, such that the only source of compartmental flow heterogeneity is the asymmetry of the bronchial tree. The model predicts expiratory flow and pressure but predictions are not dynamic or validated.

9.3.3 Summary

A review of the morphometric and mechanical models available in the literature has been presented. Single compartment models, regardless of the various regional resistances and compliances that may be incorporated, are still not able to model the effects of uneven ventilation. Multicompartmental models in the literature neglect inertance, chest wall mechanics, or a variation in mechanical properties between compartments. Thus, there exists a need for models that incorporate inertance to enable analysis at frequencies higher than typical breathing frequencies, and multiple compartments that have individual mechanical and physical properties, to better model the uneven distribution of ventilation in diseased lungs. Also, model predictions in the literature mostly represent adult values, with only a few infant models predicting overall respiratory variables. The lack of neonatal lung parameters makes it difficult to accurately quantify predictions for neonates.

9.4 MODEL DEVELOPMENT

The bronchial tree is a complex bifurcating network of airways that, according to the Weibel model [11], divides 23 times before forming millions of alveolar sacs in humans. However, when defining the different elements of the respiratory system using lumped parameter modeling, the complexity of the mathematical model can be reduced so that pressures, flows, and volumes are assumed to be uniform within well-defined control volumes. The lung can then be described as a system of branched airways, consisting of the trachea (windpipe) and bronchi (subsequent airways), leading to five chambers that represent the five separate lobes present in the actual lung. Each lobe has its own set of mechanical properties that are described in terms of elasticity, inertia, and damping elements. As a result, the model developed in this chapter is able to account for the behaviour of a five-compartment lung with differing mechanical properties and lung capacities, as well as disparities between inspiratory and expiratory airway resistances. It was not physically possible to accurately obtain empirical measurements such as pressure-volume, mass, and dimension measurements for sub-lobar segments to determine regional mechanical and physical properties within each lobe, thus restricting the current model to a maximum of five compartments. The output of the model includes airway pressures, flow rates, and volumes at the airway opening and at the individual lobes. These are used to calculate the WOB at each location as a measure of respiratory performance under different ventilation strategies.

The ovine respiratory system is modeled in this chapter. Preterm and near-term respiratory outputs can be modeled by changing the parameters to suit them. Ovine lungs are used frequently in clinical trials on neonatal respiratory mechanics, due to the similarity in size, physiological parameters, and established relationships between ovine and human gestations. Moreover, limitations on human experimentation make the ovine model an attractive alternative to investigate respiratory parameters.

The 12 airways and five lobar regions represented in the ovine respiratory system model are shown in Figure 9-16 (not to scale) and named in Table 9-1 in such a way as to reflect anatomical location.

The dynamics of the model are formulated by assuming that a uniform (but time-varying) pressure exists in each section, and that the rate of change of that pressure is dependent on the flow into and out of the section, as well as any elastic, resistive, or inertive forces present. A schematic diagram of the lumped sections of the lung is shown in Figure 9-17. The tracheo-bronchial tree, starting from the trachea, divides successively into the various secondary bronchi that lead to their respective lobes. The respective pressures and mass flow rates present in each

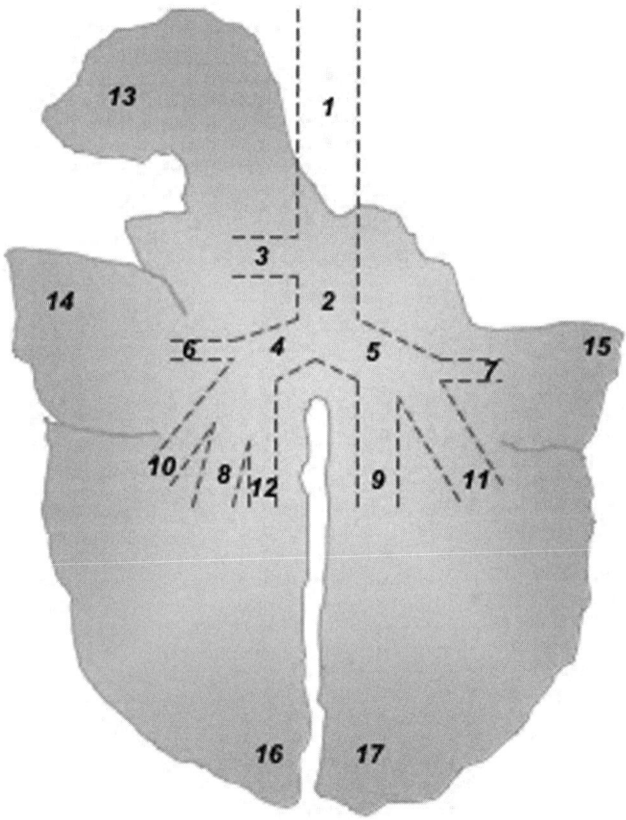

Figure 9-16. The elements of the ovine respiratory system model

section are shown in the figure and defined in more detail thereafter. The numbers correspond to those in Table 9-1.

9.4.1 Model Assumptions

- Humidity effects are neglected and all physical properties and constants are evaluated at a constant temperature of 39°C (312 K), i.e., lamb rectal temperature.
- Resistances of the airways in the lobe and the collective resistance of the lobes are assumed to be constant and the only interaction between lobes is assumed to occur at the branch points of the bronchi leading to the lobes.
- Ideal gas is assumed and gas compressibility is neglected since the Mach numbers have been calculated to be <0.2 for typical flows in all airways.

TABLE 9-1. The 17 Elements of the Ovine Respiratory System Model

1 - Upper trachea
2 - Lower trachea
3 - Right apical bronchus
4 - Right main bronchus
5 - Left main bronchus
6 - Right cardiac bronchus
7 - Left cardiac bronchus
8 - Right major diaphragmatic bronchus
9 - Left major diaphragmatic bronchus
10 - Right posterior diaphragmatic bronchus
11 - Left posterior diaphragmatic bronchus
12 - Right anterior diaphragmatic bronchus
13 - Right apical lobe
14 - Right cardiac lobe
15 - Left cardiac lobe
16 - Right diaphragmatic lobe
17 - Left diaphragmatic lobe

- Lobe surface area is assumed to remain constant unlike in reality, where the area changes with lung volume. Since this relationship is uncharacterized for premature lambs, a constant surface area is assumed.
- Lobe and airway pressures are assumed to be uniform. Although in reality there are variations in pressure within the lobe, this assumption is adequate for the present level of investigation where the trends in overall differences in respiratory parameters across lobes are of consideration. Such effects can be added to the model in the future by adding more compartments to the individual lobes to account for regional pressure variations.
- The airways are assumed to be straight with constant circular cross-section. Airways can also be modeled as collapsible tubes if desired, based on the cross-sectional area-transmural pressure relationship. This relationship is undefined in the literature for premature neonatal lambs. The trachea and primary bronchi contain cartilage and some remnants of cartilage that are still present at the level of the secondary bronchi. This makes these airways more rigid than the rest of the conducting airways. Therefore, to reduce the complexity of the model and increase solver efficiency, elementary dissipative pressure losses in a bifurcating airway system are modeled as the primary pressure-loss phe-

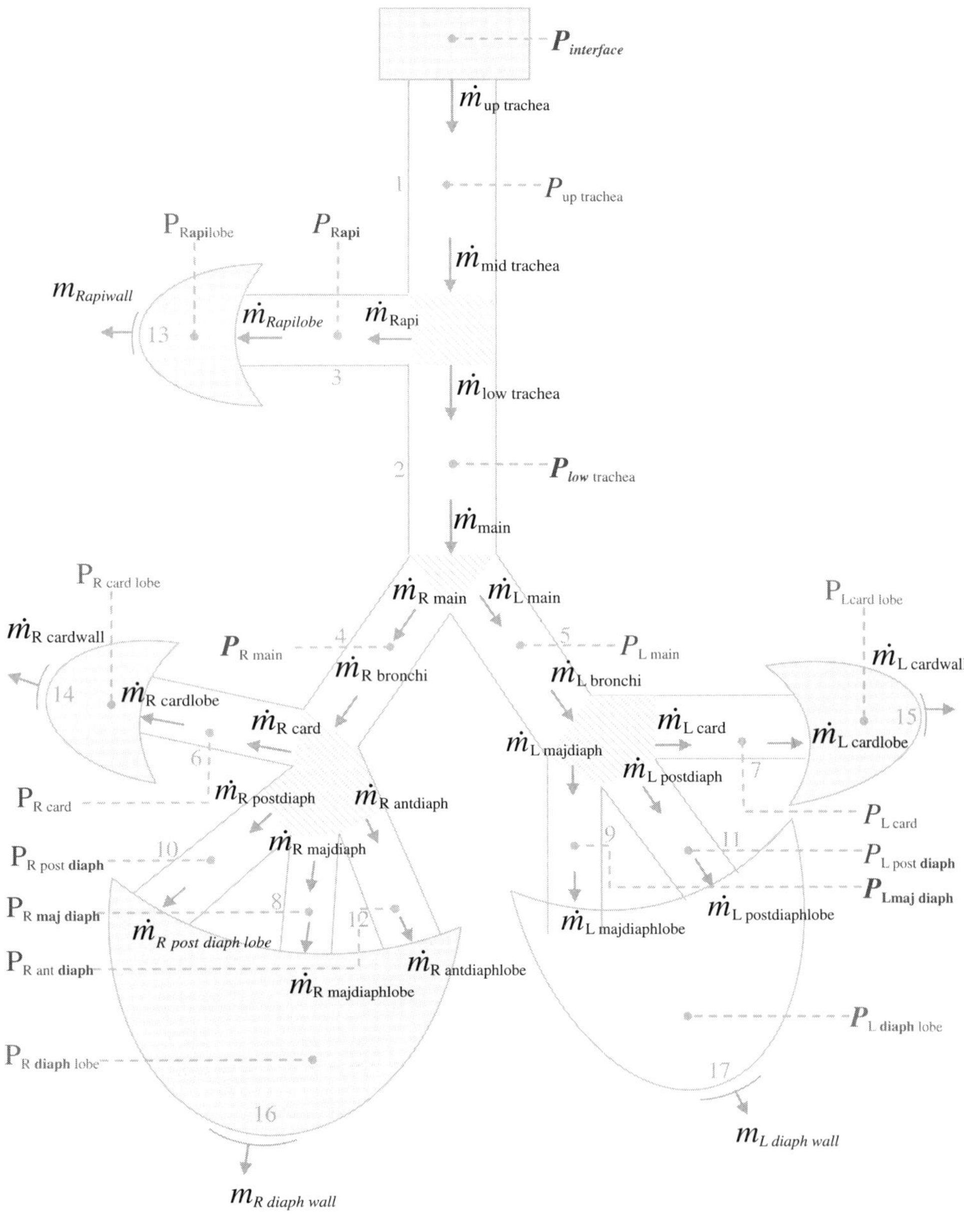

Figure 9-17. Schematic diagram of the lumped respiratory system (showing section numbering)

nomenon. However, the model retains fundamental features of airway branching, mechanical, and physical properties. It is also constructed so as to facilitate the addition of bronchial wall compliance in future studies that may be conducted in this area.

9.4.2 Model Derivation

The rate of change of pressure in sections 1 to 12 can be derived from the ideal gas equation of state.

$$P_{section}V_{section} = m_{section}RT \qquad (9-6)$$

where $P_{section}$ is the absolute pressure within the section (Pa), $V_{section}$ the volume of the section (m^3), $m_{section}$ the mass of air in the section (kg), R the specific gas constant of air at 312 K [$Pa.m^3/(kg.K)$] and T is the temperature in Kelvin (K).

If we consider a time-varying pressure in any particular section, equation (9-6) becomes:

$$\frac{d(P_{section}V_{section})}{dt} = \frac{d(m_{section}RT)}{dt} \qquad (9-7)$$

Assuming $V_{section}$, R, and T constant, equation (9-2) becomes:

$$\frac{dP_{section}}{dt} = \frac{RT}{V_{section}}\frac{dm_{section}}{dt} \qquad (9-8)$$

Applying the conservation of mass to a section gives the change in the mass of air in that section, $\Delta m_{section}$. This can be written as:

$$\Delta m_{section} = m_{in} - m_{out} \qquad (9-9)$$

where m_{in} is the mass that enters the section; and m_{out} is the mass that leaves the section. For a time-varying system,

$$\frac{dm_{section}}{dt} = \frac{d(m_{in} - m_{out})}{dt} \qquad (9-10)$$

and thus

$$\frac{dm_{section}}{dt} = \frac{d}{dt}(m_{in} - m_{out}) = \dot{m}_{in} - \dot{m}_{out} \qquad (9-11)$$

Equation (9-8) can now be written as

$$\frac{dP_{section}}{dt} = \frac{RT}{V_{section}}(\dot{m}_{in} - \dot{m}_{out}) \qquad (9-12)$$

For regions 13 to 17 (the lobes), where the volume of the region varies with time, equation (9-8) changes to:

$$\frac{d(P_{lobe}V_{lobe})}{dt} = \frac{dm_{lobe}}{dt}RT \qquad (9-13)$$

which can be expanded to the following form:

$$\frac{dP_{lobe}}{dt}V_{lobe} + \frac{dV_{lobe}}{dt}P_{lobe} = (\dot{m}_{in} - \dot{m}_{out})RT \qquad (9-14)$$

Equations (9-12) and (9-14) can be used to obtain expressions of the pressure in the individual airway segments and lobes, respectively. The mass flow rates and pressures involved are those presented in Figure 9-17.

9.4.3 Mass Flow Rate Expressions

Thus far, the mass flow rates in the derivation represent the mass flow at specific points, i.e., at the boundaries of each section. The walls in sections 1 to 12 contain varying amounts of cartilage and so may be considered to be vastly more rigid than subsequent airways. In order to simplify the model for the purposes of this study, sections 1 to 12 are assumed to be rigid.

This implies that there is no variation in mass in sections 1 to 12. The sections are also very short (in the order of a few centimeters), such that any pressure variations within the section are very small and can be ignored. It can thus be assumed that the pressure at each boundary is equal to the pressure in the section that is situated upwind from that boundary.

In the simplest case, mass flow rate can be determined by the pressure-flow characteristics as described by Poiseuille's equation for laminar flow in straight, circular tubes. However, the mass flow rate in a monopodial branching network can be more accurately determined by empirical relations developed by Reynolds and Lee [24], where the total pressure loss in a canine airway segment ΔP_{total} was found to be related to the flow rate and its square for Reynolds numbers tested up to 10,000. The following calculations show how the Reynolds-Lee equations [24] can be used to describe the inspiratory and expiratory mass flows in the tracheal and bronchial segments, as a function of Poiseuille pressure drop across that segment ($\Delta P_{Poiseuille}$) and the Reynolds Number (Re).

Reynolds and Lee describe their data using a dimensionless Rohrer equation:

$$\Delta P_{total} = (a + b\,\mathrm{Re})\Delta P_{poiseuille} \qquad (9-15)$$

TABLE 9-2. Scaling factors in Reynolds-Lee equation [24]

	Inspiration		Expiration	
	a	*b*	*a*	*b*
Tracheal segments	24	0.0162	50	0.0162
All airways below trachea	15	0.0146	40	0.0116

where a and b are scaling coefficients as defined by Reynolds and Lee, and are listed in Table 9-2 for the trachea and subsequent airways. The values of a are much larger for expiration than for inspiration for a given airway, meaning that static pressure drop is much larger for expiration than inspiration. The values for b remain similar for both inspiration and expiration in a particular airway. Reynolds and Lee attribute the increased loss in pressure during expiration to the effects of the bifurcations preceding tracheal flow as air travels up from the smaller airways, out to the airway opening.

The static pressure drop across the section $\Delta P_{section}$ can be expressed as:

$$\Delta P_{section} = P_{upwind} - P_{section} = (a + b\ \mathrm{Re})\Delta P_{poiseuille} \qquad (9-16)$$

where P_{upwind} is the pressure on the upwind boundary and

$$\Delta P_{poiseuille} = \frac{128\mu L_{section}}{\pi D_{section}{}^{4}\rho}\dot{m}_{section} \qquad (9-17)$$

In equation (9-17), $L_{section}$ and $D_{section}$ are the length and diameter of the section, respectively; $\dot{m}_{section}$ is the mass flow through the section; and μ and ρ are the dynamic viscosity and density of the air at 312.5 K.

Combining equations (9-16) and (9-17) and solving for the mass flow rate gives:

$$\dot{m}_{in} = \frac{\Delta P_{section}}{(a + bRe)}\frac{\pi D_{section}{}^{4}\rho}{128\mu L_{section}} \qquad (9-18)$$

Substituting values for a and b for each respective airway produces expressions for the individual airway segments (sections 1 to 12).

The mass flow rates that enter the lobes are dependent on the conductance of the individual lobes and the difference in pressure between the lobe and the section preceding it. Values for the total conductance of the airways that make up the individual lobes are assumed to be constants. The mass flow rate into a particular lobe may be expressed as

$$\dot{m}_{in} = (P_{section} - P_{lobe}) \times C_{lobe} \qquad (9-19)$$

9.4.4 Lobe Dynamics

Assumptions and Justifications: The five-lobe model presented in this section is well suited to describe the uneven distribution of ventilation across the lobes, and the inhomogeneities in neonatal lung mechanics. The consideration of the different properties of each lobe increases the number of parameters significantly. So far, the practical value of such a model for simulation studies in premature neonates is limited because a great number of reference values and parameters are unknown. However, various parameters collected by Reddy [25] for a premature ovine lung required for the model were through experiments and calculations based on reference values from the literature.

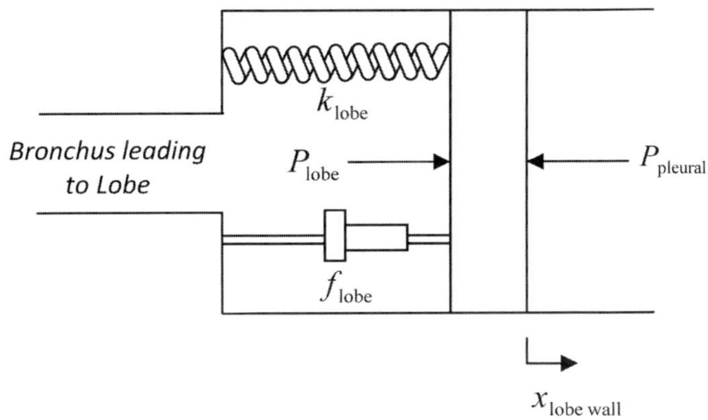

Figure 9-18. General schematic for a lobe spring mass damper system

A mechanical model that allows direct substitution of most measured parameters is used to describe the mechanics of each lobe. The concept of a moving piston of a mass M_{lobe} forms the basis of the model. It accounts for the motion of the lobe wall and the gas flow effects. A variable spring stiffness (k_{lobe}) describes the elastic properties of the lobe and a constant viscous resistance (f_{lobe}) describes the viscous resistance of the lung tissue. The inertive, elastic, and viscous forces caused by these elements act on the piston (lobe) area (A_{lobe}), which is equivalent to the lobe wall. The piston is subject to the pressure in the lobe (P_{lobe}) and the pleural pressure ($P_{pleural}$). Lobe pressures are assumed to be uniform and the area of the piston remains constant, although in reality there are variations in pressure within the lobe, and the surface area of the lobe changes with a change in volume (changing the predicted pressures in the lobe). Such effects can be added to the model in the future by adding more compartments to the individual lobes to account for regional pressure variations, and by determining the surface area-lung volume relationship to account for the changing surface area.

Derivation: A general form of the equation of motion is derived based on the schematic diagram in Figure 9-18. Applying Newton's second law, the equation of motion for the lobe wall can be written as:

$$-k_{lobe}x_{lobe\ wall} - f_{lobe}\frac{dx_{lobe\ wall}}{dt} + (P_{lobe} - P_{pleural})A_{lobe} = M_{lobe}\frac{d^2x_{lobe\ wall}}{dt^2} \quad (9-20)$$

where $\frac{d^2x_{lobe\ wall}}{dt^2}$, $\frac{dx_{lobe\ wall}}{dt}$, and $x_{lobe\ wall}$ are the acceleration, velocity, and displacement of the lobe wall, respectively.

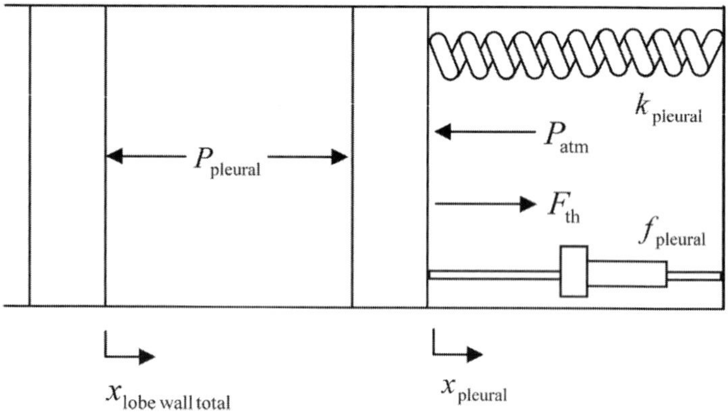

Figure 9-19. Schematic of pleural compartment and chest wall

The mass flow rate of air caused by the motion of the lobe wall may be expressed as:

$$\dot{m}_{lobe\ wall} = \rho A_{lobe} \frac{dx_{lobe\ wall}}{dt} \qquad (9-21)$$

where ρ is the air density at 312.5 K. The lobe volume (V_{lobe}) is regarded as a control volume, which is determined from the displacement of the lobe wall ($x_{\text{lobe wall}}$) multiplied by the piston surface area (A_{lobe}), such that:

$$V_{lobe} = A_{lobe} x_{lobe\ wall} \qquad (9-22)$$

Using equations (9-20) to (9-22), the equivalent expressions for each individual lobe can be obtained.

9.4.5 The Pleural Compartment and Chest Wall

Assumptions and Simplifications: The pleural compartment is modeled along lines similar to those of lobes, as seen in Figure 9-19. However, it has two notable differences: (1) there is no airflow into or out of the compartment; and (2) it is a closed compartment that is filled with pleural liquid (instead of air as in the lung).

An equivalent variable stiffness ($k_{pleural}$) is assumed to represent the elastic properties of the rib cage, diaphragm, and pleural fluid and tissue. Also, these properties generate an equivalent viscous resistance ($f_{pleural}$), which is assumed to act on the pleural wall of an equivalent surface area $A_{pleural}$. The combined movement of the lobe walls ($x_{\text{lobe wall total}}$) is the sum of $x_{R\ api\ wall}$, $x_{R\ card\ wall}$, $x_{R\ diaph\ wall}$, $x_{L\ card\ wall}$, and $x_{L\ diaph\ wall}$. The pleural compartment experiences forces generated by the pleural pressure ($P_{pleural}$), atmospheric pressure (P_{atm}), and the thoracic force (F_{th}). These forces act to change the volume of the compartment. F_{th} is the force generated by the rib cage and diaphragm muscles due to the neurogenic signals sent by the brain, to drive lung motion and hence create the tidal volume. It is the main driving force of the model and idealized as acting on a single point of the pleural surface. It is commonly defined as a signal with a profile that follows the shape (but not the magnitude) of the tidal volume [20].

In reality, the situation is far more complex with the force adapting itself to respond to the changing levels of oxygen and carbon dioxide in the blood stream. The physiological aspects of gas exchange can be introduced into the model through additional subsystems that account for gas diffusion at the alveolar level, the partial pressures of oxygen in the bloodstream, and the resulting neural control of breathing. These elements, however, are out of the scope of this research, which concentrates purely on the mechanical aspects of respiration.

In normal adult respiration, regional variations in pleural pressure exist due to the downward-acting weight forces of the lung. However, since neonatal subjects receiving respiratory support are never upright, the regional differences in pleural pressure are much less significant and so can be ignored for the purposes of this model.

Derivation: Using Newton's second law, the equation of motion of the pleural wall is:

$$F_{\text{th}} - k_{pleural} x_{pleural} - f_{pleural} \frac{dx_{pleural}}{dt} + (P_{pleural} - P_{atm}) A_{pleural} = M_{pleural} \frac{d^2 x_{pleural}}{dt^2} \qquad (9-23)$$

where M_{pleural} is the mass of the moving part of the chest wall; and $\frac{d^2 x_{pleural}}{dt^2}$, $\frac{dx_{pleural}}{dt}$, and $x_{pleural}$ are the acceleration, velocity, and displacement of the pleural wall, respectively.

Since the fluid inside the pleural compartment is liquid, the rate of change of the pleural pressure depends on the expansion and compression of the pleural fluid, and may be derived by using the effective bulk modulus ($B_{pleural}$). By definition:

$$B_{pleural} = \frac{\dfrac{dP_{pleural}}{dt}}{\left(\dfrac{dV_{pleural}}{dt}\right) \Big/ V_{pleural}} \qquad (9-24)$$

Rearranging, gives:

$$\frac{dP_{pleural}}{dt} = \frac{B_{pleural}}{V_{pleural}} \left(\frac{dV_{pleural}}{dt} \right) \qquad (9-25)$$

The change in the pleural compartment volume $\left(\frac{dV_{pleural}}{dt}\right)$ is determined by the displacement of the pleural and lobe walls, and so equation (9-25) is expanded to give:

$$\frac{dP_{pleural}}{dt} = \frac{B_{pleural}}{V_{pleural}} \begin{bmatrix} A_{pleural}\frac{dx_{pleural}}{dt} - A_{\mathrm{R}\ api}\frac{dx_{\mathrm{R}\ api\ wall}}{dt} - A_{\mathrm{R}\ card}\frac{dx_{\mathrm{R}\ card\ wall}}{dt} \\ A_{\mathrm{R}\ diaph}\frac{dx_{\mathrm{R}\ diaph\ wall}}{dt} - A_{L\ card}\frac{dx_{\mathrm{L}\ card\ wall}}{dt} - A_{L\ diaph}\frac{dx_{L\ diaph\ wall}}{dt} \end{bmatrix} \quad (9-26)$$

9.5 SIMULINK™ MODEL

A Simulink™ model is formulated for a 128-day (preterm) gestation lamb. The Simulink™ model includes look-up tables, which contain input and output numeric values to describe the relationship between elastance and lobe volume for each lobe. Since these relationships are different at each lobe and at each gestation, two separate models are created.

The model is able to predict the pressure, flow rate, and volume at each of the 17 sections identified in Table 9-1. Figure 9-20 shows the three main subsystems of the model within the Simulink™ environment, i.e., the tracheobronchial subsystem, the viscoelastic subsystem, and the respiratory support device subsystem. Each subsystem is a modular, connectable subroutine (consisting of many smaller subroutines) based on the equations derived in this chapter.

Figure 9-21 shows the general form of the block diagrams in the tracheobronchial system, using the general forms in equations (9-12) and (9-18). This arrangement constitutes the subsystems in the model that calculate the mass flow rates and pressures in each airway section.

Figure 9-22 shows the general form of the block diagrams in the viscoelastic system, using the general forms in equations (9-14) and (9-19). This arrangement constitutes the subsystems in the model that calculate the pressures in each lobe and the mass flow rates into the lobes from the connecting airway sections.

Figure 9-23 shows the general form of the block diagrams used for the general forms of equations (9-20) to (9-22). This arrangement constitutes the subsystems in the model that calculate the individual lobe wall movements due to the various forces acting on the lobe walls, and hence the mass flow rate generated by each lobe due to patient breathing.

Figure 9-24 shows the block diagram for equation (9-23) in the viscoelastic system. This arrangement constitutes the subsystem in the model that calculates the movement of the pleural wall due to the forces that act on it.

Figure 9-25 shows the block diagram for equation (9-26) in the viscoelastic system. This arrangement constitutes the subsystem in the

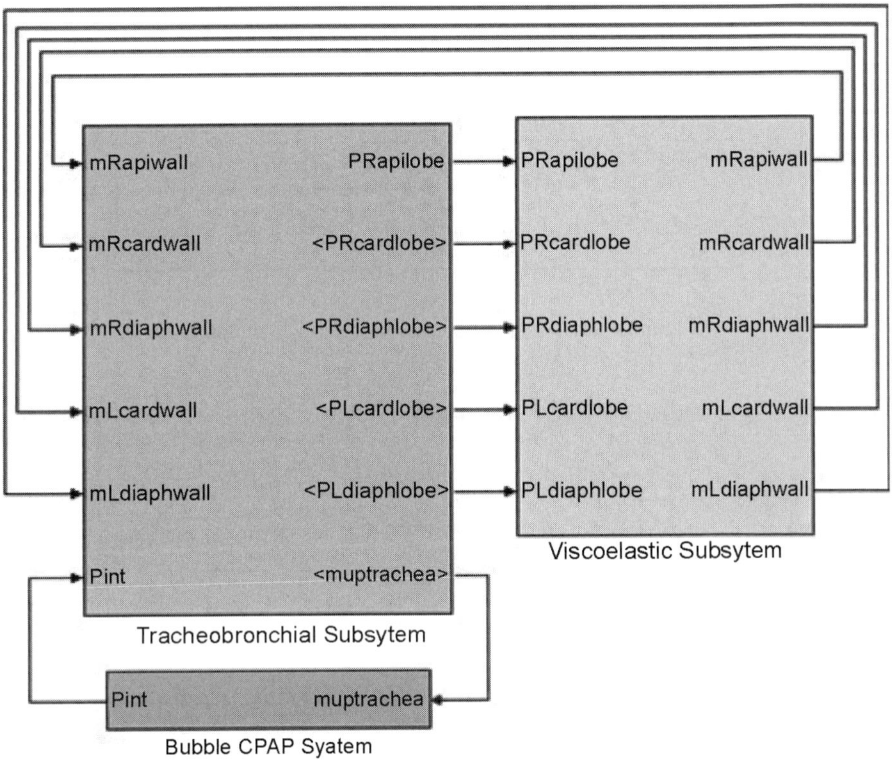

Figure 9-20. Elements of the Simulink™ model

model that calculates the pleural pressure, which acts on the wall of the individual lobes.

The respiratory support device subsystem is the Simulink™ model developed in Chapter 8 [26], which models the Bubble CPAP device. The patient mass flow rate ($\dot{m}_{up\ trachea}$) flows into the patient interface of the Bubble CPAP device and contributes to the pressure generated at the

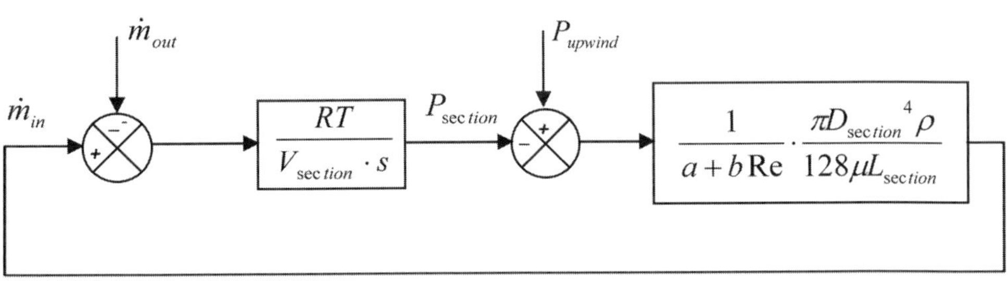

Figure 9-21. General form of the block diagram for equations (9-12) and (9-18)

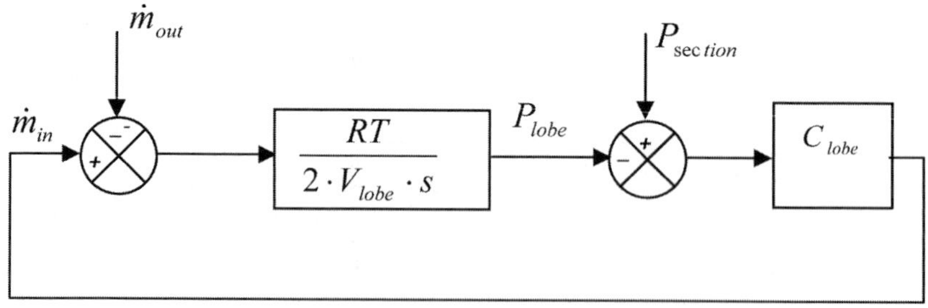

Figure 9-22. General form for the block diagram for equations (9-14) and (9-19)

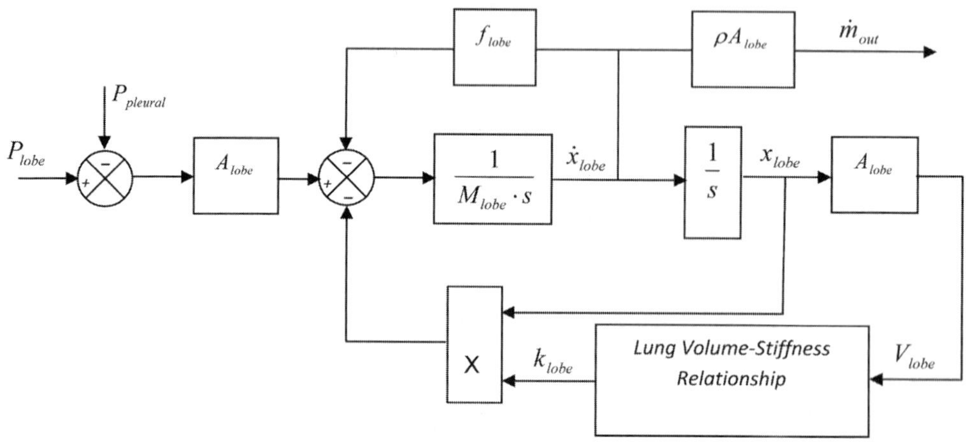

Figure 9-23. General form for the block diagram for equations (9-20) to (9-22)

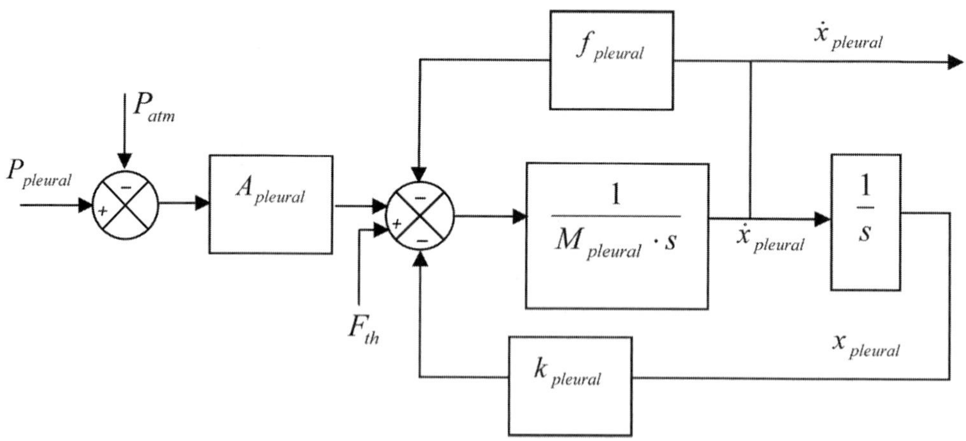

Figure 9-24. Block diagram for equation (9-23)

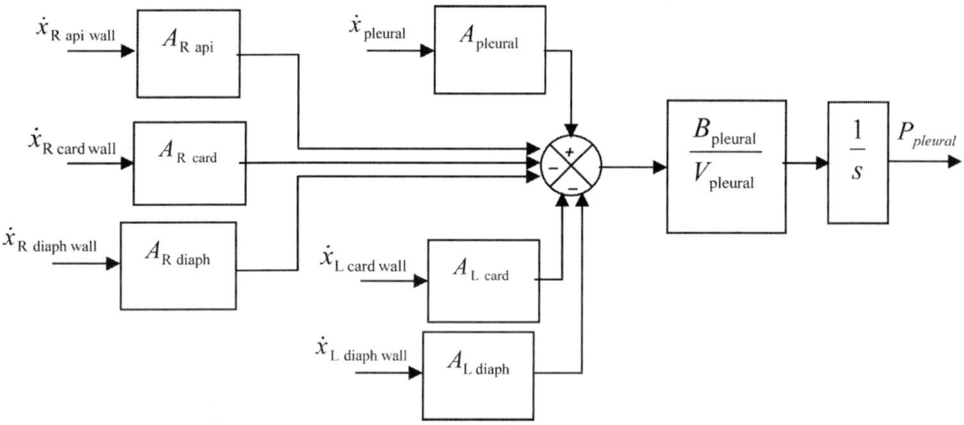

Figure 9-25. Block diagram for equation (9-26)

interface ($P_{interface}$), which in turn acts on the upper trachea as in equation (9-18). The Bubble CPAP System can be substituted for any other model of a respiratory device (i.e. CPAP, HFV, MV, etc.)

The parameters for the model are stored in a Matlab m-file, which is loaded before performing any simulation. Desired outputs (i.e., pressure, flow rate, and volume) are obtained by placing scopes in the desired locations (i.e., sections 1 and 13 to 17), which log the data into arrays in the Matlab workspace.

The sample time for all simulations is 0.004 seconds (250 Hz) since frequencies up to 125 Hz were used. The "ode23s" variable-step continuous

TABLE 9-3. Airway lengths and diameters

	Measurement/Birth Weight, mm/kg (±SD)	
Airway Number and Description	**Length**	**Diameter**
1 - Upper trachea	37.11 (2.72)	2.64 (0.20)
2 - Lower trachea	8.85 (1.10)	2.48 (0.24)
3 - Right apical bronchus	2.48 (0.38)	2.35 (0.27)
4 - Right main bronchus	3.59 (0.40)	2.29 (0.27)
5 - Left main bronchus	1.74 (0.30)	2.21 (0.29)
6 - Right cardiac bronchus	2.08 (0.36)	2.16 (0.31)
7 - Left cardiac bronchus	1.99 (0.27)	1.36 (0.16)
8 - Right major diaphragmatic bronchus	2.83 (0.47)	1.03 (0.13)
9 - Left major diaphragmatic bronchus	2.25 (0.31)	1.08 (0.21)
10 - Right posterior diaphragmatic bronchus	1.56 (0.32)	0.84 (0.18)
11 - Left posterior diaphragmatic bronchus	2.88 (0.40)	0.84 (0.11)
12 - Right anterior diaphragmatic bronchus	1.75 (0.23)	0.89 (0.11)

TABLE 9-4. Preterm lung properties

	Average Mass g/kg (±SD)	Surface Area m^2/kg	Volume mL/kg	Conductance [(kg/s)/Pa]/kg
Chest wall	74.83(6.82)	-	-	-
Total lung	29.30(2.37)	-	-	-
Left lung	12.45(1.14)	-	-	-
Right lung	16.85(1.43)	-	-	-
Right apical lobe	4.02(0.84)	0.32	1.17	8.77E-09
Right cardiac lobe	2.64(0.42)	0.21	0.78	5.82E-09
Right diaphragmatic lobe	10.19(0.84)	0.80	2.99	2.24E-08
Left cardiac lobe	3.95(0.48)	0.31	1.15	8.64E-09
Left daphragmatic lobe	8.51(0.72)	0.67	2.50	1.87E-08

solver in Simulink™ is used here. It computes the model's state at the next time step using a modified Rosenbrock formula of the order 2. It is a one-step solver, needing only the solution to the preceding time point. It shows more efficiency at the crude tolerances that were used in the simulation.

Parameters required for the model are vast and obtained from experimentation and estimations from the literature. The values are briefly presented here. The average airway lengths and diameters measured from eight lung casts are given in Table 9-3 [25]. The lobe masses measured from eight lungs [25], as well as estimated surface areas, volumes [27-29], and conductance's [30, 31] are given in Table 9-4. The elastance of the lobes is defined by the relationship given by Venegas et al. [32], which uses pressure-volume data measured from eight lungs. The fitting parameters for the relationship that represents the premature lamb lung are given in Table 9-5.

9.6 MODEL VALIDATION

We have modeled the Bubble CPAP device in Chapter 8 as an application of the "Talkative Models" approach. This model will be incorporated

TABLE 9-5. Fitting parameters for elastance relationships

	Right Apical	Right Cardiac	Right Diaphragmatic	Left Cardiac	Left Diaphragmatic
a	-288.30	-288.56	-287.90	-288.62	-288.17
b	289.54	289.38	291.05	289.84	290.81
c	-69.69	-74.96	-57.62	-70.03	-59.95
d	12.67	12.68	12.63	12.69	12.64
R^2	0.997	0.997	0.997	0.997	0.997

into the lung model developed in this chapter to determine the interaction between the lung and the device for RDS treatment.

In order to validate the model, the pressure, flow, and volume at the airway opening of 133-day gestation lambs (closest available results to 128-day gestation) receiving CPAP with a bias flow of 8 L/min (n=12) are obtained from the study by Pillow et al. [33]. Data from one animal, which has the tidal volume closest to the average tidal volume of the sample population and so displays typical measurements of pressure, flow, and tidal volume, is selected for comparison (details shown in Table 9-6). The animal-specific parameters in the 128-day gestation model are set to those of Table 9-6.

The resulting model predictions at the airway opening of volume, airway pressure, and flow are shown in Figure 9-26 (a) to (c), respectively, and show a close correlation with experimental results. The deviation of the model results from the experimental results is quantified as a percentage difference with respect to the experimental results at the points of maximum, minimum, and mean pressure and flow (Table 9-7), showing a maximum of 11% deviation from the experimentally measured respiratory parameters.

The respiratory variables of a subject receiving Bubble CPAP are also predicted at the airway opening. As done previously with the lambs on CPAP, typical pressure, flow, and volume at the airway opening of 133-day gestation lambs receiving Bubble CPAP with a bias flow of 8 L/min (n=12) are also obtained from the study by Pillow et al. [33]. The animal-specific parameters in the model are adjusted to those of the selected animal described in Table 9-6. All other parameters and settings are left unchanged. In addition to the prescribed level of mean CPAP (6.75 cm H_2O) as used in the initial simulation, a typical signal of the superimposed pressure oscillations generated at the level of the CPAP generator of the Bubble CPAP system is introduced into the model by using the model developed in Chapter 8. The model predictions and comparative experimental data are shown in Figure 9-26.

Overall, the model predictions show good comparisons with experimental data. The superimposed pressure oscillations are clearly visible in Figure 9-26 (d) and (e). Because of the random nature of the bubble oscillations, the experimental and model values do not match exactly but lie in the same pressure range. The tidal volume values during Bubble CPAP (Figure 9-26 (f)) show some unevenness in profile due to the pressure oscillations, which are not as distinct as those seen in the pressure and flow

TABLE 9.6. Details of selected animals on CPAP and bubble CPAP

Treatment Type	CPAP	Bubble CPAP
Birth weight (kg)	3.15	3.2
Tidal Volume (mL/kg)	4.76	4.94
Respiratory rate (breaths/min)	60	98
Mean CPAP (cmH_2O)	6.75	6.75

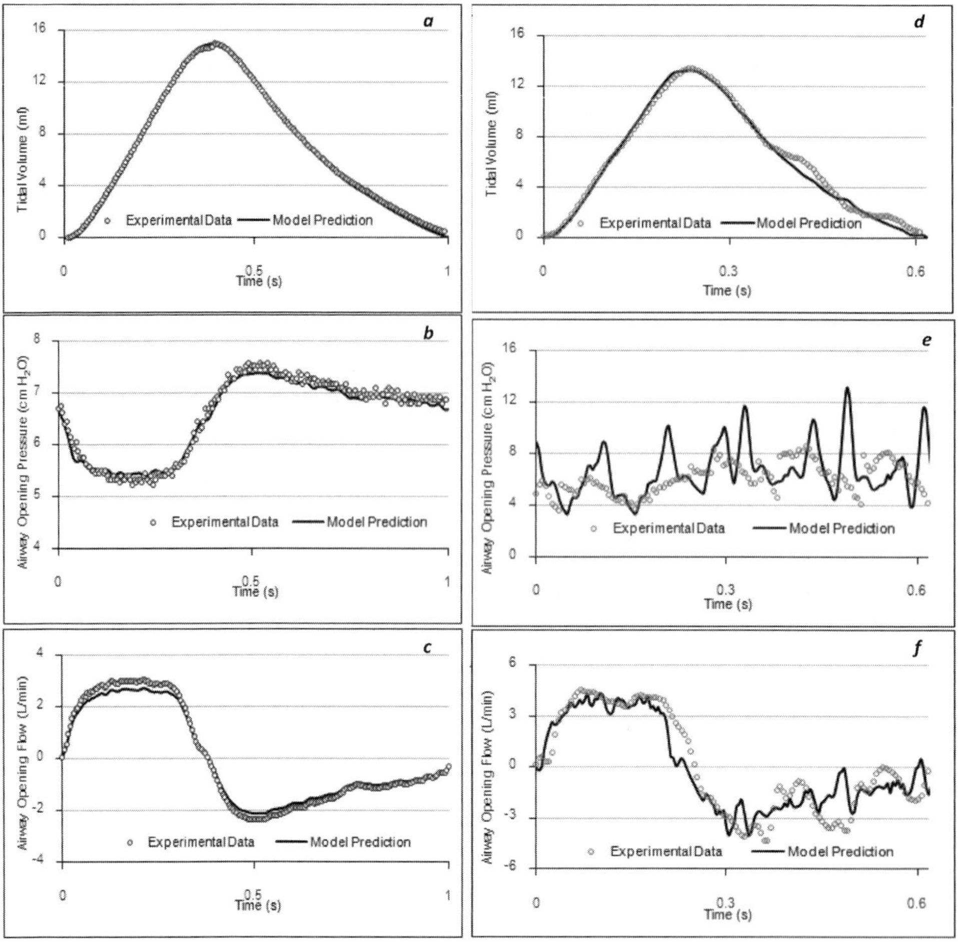

Figure 9-26. Model-experiment comparison of a preterm lamb on CPAP (a-c) and bubble CPAP (d-f)

profiles. The tidal volume is calculated in the model (as well as measured in clinical practice) by the mathematical integration of the flow signal.

The oscillation in the experimental values appears to be slightly more "damped" than the model predictions. This may be because the fittings at the patient interface in the experiment may have been adapted

TABLE 9-7. Model-experiment percentage difference in respiratory variables

Percent Difference in Pressure			Percent Difference Flow		
Max	*Mean*	*Min*	*Max*	*Mean*	*Min*
2.36	4.95	10.6	11.0	0.68	10.5

slightly to incorporate the endotracheal tube and attachments. Also, the model does not account for leaks and shock factors due to fittings in the system, preserving the pressure oscillation frequencies and amplitudes to a greater extent than in real life.

9.7 PREDICTIONS OF PRESSURE OSCILLATION TRANSMISSION THROUGH THE TRACHEOBRONCHIAL TREE

It has often been questioned in practice whether the pressure oscillations produced by the Bubble CPAP system actually reach the level of the lobes. Since in-vivo measurements at the level of the lobes remains impractical at present, the model can be used to give some insight into such behavior. Figure 9-27 shows how the model can be used for such purposes. It shows the volume, pressure, and flow predictions in each lobe.

The oscillations in pressure and flow are visible at the level of the individual lobes. The magnitude of the pressure oscillations in Figure 9-27 (a) and (b) are not markedly decreased compared with those at the interface. The magnitude of the flow oscillations in Figure 9-27 (c) and (d) show a decrease in magnitude compared with those at the interface. Again, the volumes in the lobes (Figure 9-27 (e) and (f)) show no noticeable change in profile with the addition of oscillations.

The absence of attenuation in pressure oscillations may be due to the airways being modeled as rigid tubes. In reality, the first few generations of airways, although they do contain cartilage, are not completely rigid and do have some compliance that will dampen the amplitude and frequencies of oscillations traveling through them. By defining the airway pressure cross-sectional area or volume relationship in the airways, it is possible to achieve a more accurate model of the airway pressure drop. However, to accurately determine these relationships requires detailed empirical measurements on the fragile ovine airways, which were beyond the scope of this research and remain a subject of further study. Lambert et al. [34] developed airway pressure cross-sectional area relationships for airways, and these were used by Polak and Lutchen [23] to describe the mechanical characteristics of the airways. However, these relationships were developed from a symmetrical Weibel model [11] for adult human lungs for expiratory flow only, and any relationships deduced for neonates would be scaled down by lung volume and thus less accurate.

The oscillations in flow rate (Figure 9-27 (c) and (d)) are still visible at the level of the lobes and although they may decrease in absolute amplitude due to the division of flow across the lobes, they do not decrease relative to the maximum flow rate value in each lobe. This may be attributed to the fact that the mechanical properties of each lobe are more

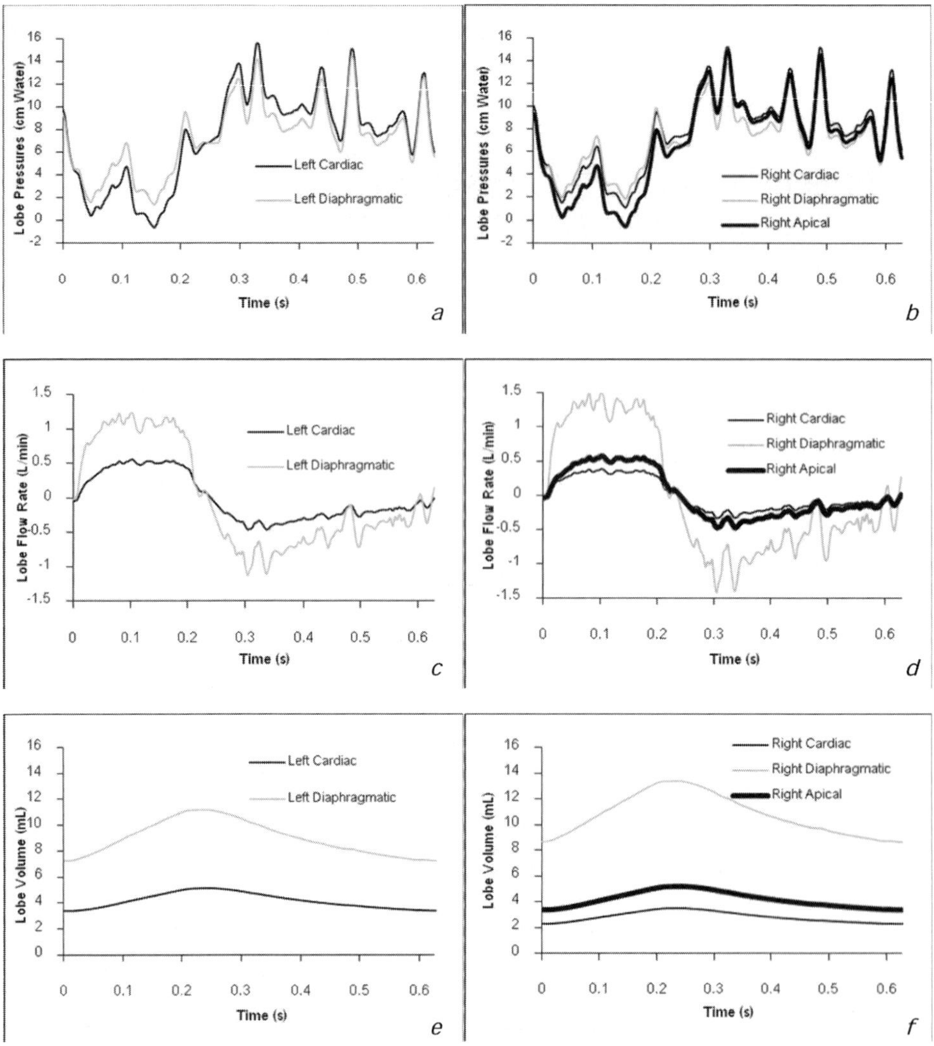

Figure 9-27. Predictions of respiratory parameters at the lobes

or less homogeneous when corrected for the maximum volume per birth weight, which was used to determine the stiffness-volume relationship in each lobe based on the pressure-volume curve of the whole lung.

A more heterogeneous description of the pressure-volume relationship of each lobe will represent a more diseased state, and hence show oscillations in pressure and flow rate of different frequencies and amplitudes. Also, with the correction in the description of the airway pressure calculations, the amplitudes of the oscillations in flow rate will also decrease.

Figure 9-27 (e) and (f) clearly indicate that the tidal volume calculations show no significant pressure oscillations due to the integration process.

9.8 CLOSURE

This chapter systematically introduces the reader to a simplified approach of dealing with the complexities of modeling a non-linear biological system such as the lung. A lumped parameter model of the tracheobronchial tree and the viscoelastice components of the respiratory system are presented, and it is illustrated how such a model can be used as an example of the "Talkative Models" approach introduced in Chapter 1.

REFERENCES

[1] Ganong, W.F., Review of Medical Physiology. 2001, New York: McGraw-Hill.

[2] Gray, H., Gray's Anatomy of the Human Body. 2000, Philedelphia: Lea and Febiger, 1918.

[3] Marieb, E.N., Mallat, J., Wilhelm, P.B., Human Anatomy. 5th ed. 2008, San Francisco: Benjamin Cummings.

[4] Polin, R.A. and W.W. Fox, Fetal and Neonatal Physiology. 2nd ed. 1997, Philadelphia: WB Saunders Co.

[5] West, J.B., Respiratory Physiology. The Essentials. 6th ed. 2000, Baltimore: Lippincott Williams and Wilkins.

[6] De Jongh, F., Ventilation Modelling of the Human Lung, in Faculty of Aerospace Engineering. 1995, Delft University of Technology: Delft. p. 197.

[7] Goldsmith, J.P. and E.H. Karotkin, Assisted Ventilation of the Neonate. 2003, Philadelphia: Saunders.

[8] Hall, S.B., et al., Approximations in the measurement of surface tension on the oscillating bubble surfactometer. *American Physiological Society*, 1993. **75**(1): p. 468–477.

[9] ATS/ERS Statement on Respiratory Muscle Testing. *Am J Respir Crit Care Med*, 2002. **166**: p. 518–624.

[10] Crimer, G.J., et al., Critical Care Study Guide. 2002, Philadelphia: Springer.

[11] Weibel, E.R., Morphometry of the human lung. 1963, New York: Academic Press: Springer-Verlag.

[12] Hansen, J.E. and E.P. Ampaya, Human air space shapes, sizes, areas, volumes. *J Appl Physiol*, 1975. **38**(6): p. 990–995.

[13] Horsfield, K., et al., Models of the human bronchial tree. *J Appl Physiol*, 1971. **31**(2): p. 207–217.

[14] Tawhai, M.H., K.S. Burrowes, and E.A. Hoffman, Computational models of structure-function relationships in the pulmonary circulation and their validation. *Exp Physiol*, 2006. **91**(2): p. 285–293.

[15] Woo, T., et al. A comparison of various respiratory system models based on parameter estimates from impulse oscillometry data. in Proc 26th Annual Conf IEEE EMBS. 2004. San Francisco.

[16] Schmidt, M., et al., Computer simulation of the measured respiratory impedance in newborn infants and the effect of the measurement equipment. *Medical Engineering and Physics*, 1998. **20**: p. 220–228.

[17] Mead, J., Mechanical properties of the lung. *Physiol Rev*, 1961. **41**: p. 281–320.

[18] Athanasiades, A., et al., Energy analysis of a nonlinear model of the normal lung. *Journal of Biological Systems*, 2000. **8**(2): p. 115–139.

[19] Liu, C.H., et al., Airway mechanics, gas exchange and blood flow in a nonlinear model of the normal human lung. *J Appl Physiol*, 1998. **84**: p. 1447–1469.

[20] Tomlinson, S.P., D.G. Tilley, and C.R. Burrows, Computer simulation of human interaction with underwater breathing equipment. *Journal of Engineering in Medicine*, 1994. **208**: p. 249–261.

[21] Crooke, P.S. and J.D. Head, A general two-compartment model for mechanical ventilation. *Mathl Comput Modeling*, 1996. **24**(7): p. 1–18.

[22] Bates, J.H.T. and J. Milic-Emili, Influence of the viscoelastic properties of the respiratory system on the energetically optimum breathing frequency. *Annals of Biomedical Engineering*, 1993. **21**: p. 489–499.

[23] Polak, A.G. and K.R. Lutchen, Computational model for forced expiration from asymmetric normal lungs. *Annals of Biomedical Engineering*, 2003. **31**(8): p. 891–907.

[24] Reynolds, D.B. and J.-S. Lee, Steady pressure-flow relationship of a model of the canine bronchial tree. *Journal of Applied Physiology*, 1981. **51**(5): p. 1072–1079.

[25] Reddy, P.I., The Effect of Pressure Oscillations on Respiratory Performance., in School of Engineering. 2009, Auckland University of Technology: Auckland. p. 226.

[26] Manilal, P., The Effect of Pressure Oscillations on Neonatal Breathing, Master of Engineering Thesis, in Diagnostics and Control Research Centre. 2004, Auckland University of Technology: Auckland. p. 134.

[27] Ashrafi, M., Jamshidi, M., Fareed, M., Sanei, M.H., Analysis of lamb lung development with tracheal ligation in left posterolateral diaphragmatic hernia in cases and controls. *Journal of Research in Medical Sciences*, 2006. **11**(5): p. 319–324.

[28] Lipsett, J., Tamblyn, M., Madigan, K., Roberts, P., Cool, J.C., Runciman, S.I., McMillen, I.C., Robinson, J., Owens, J.A., Restricted fetal growth and lung development: A morphometric analysis of pulmonary structure. *Pediatric Pulmonology*, 2006. **41**(12): p. 1138–1145.

[29] Ting, A., et al., Alveolar Vascularization of the Lung in a Lamb Model of Congenital Diaphragmatic Hernia. *Am. J. Respir. Crit. Care Med.*, 1998. **157**(1): p. 31–34.

[30] Ashgarian, B. and O.T. Price, Airflow Distribution in the Human Lung and its Influence on Particle Deposition. *Inhalation Toxicology*, 2006. **18**: p. 795–801.

[31] Kobayashi, H., et al., Estimation of the Distribution Profile of Airway Resistance in the Lungs. *Computers and Biomedical Research*, 1987. **20**: p. 507–525.

[32] Venegas, J.G., R.S. Harris, and B.A. Simon, A comprehensive equation for the pulmonary pressure-volume curve. *Journal of Applied Physiology*, 1998. **84**(1): p. 389–395.

[33] Pillow, J., et al., Bubble Continuous Positive Airway Pressure Enhances Lung Volume and Gas Exchange in Preterm Lambs. *Am. J. Respir. Crit. Care Med.*, 2007. **176**: p. 63–69.

[34] Lambert, R.K., Wilson, T. A.,Hyatt, R. E.,Rodarte, J. R., A computational model for expiratory flow. *J Appl Physiol*, 1982. **52**(1): p. 44–56.

Appendix A

CPAP AIR DELIVERY

The main purpose of the air delivery unit (ADU) is to provide a patient suffering from Obstructive Sleep Apnea (OSA) with the required output pressure for effective treatment. Compressors can be classified into Positive Type and Non-positive Type air compressors.

A.1 POSITIVE TYPE AIR COMPRESSORS

Positive displacement compressors, such as reciprocating and rocking piston, rotary vane, rotary screw, and lobed rotor are ideal for achieving very high air pressures and mass flow rates without the need for high operational speeds. However, contamination of the breathing air through oil or carbon particles is a significant problem encountered in most of these compressor types. Despite refinement in seal quality and the use of metallic coatings to reduce friction, there is still a lubrication requirement, and oil carry-over into the air stream is still a problem [1]. The Diaphragm type positive displacement compressor avoids these problems by utilizing a thin elastic diaphragm, eliminating the need for piston or compressor scroll lubrication. It isolates the airflow from the operational mechanism if desired and seems a good option for the breathing system under consideration. In spite of the fact that these types of compressor could be used in a Continuous Positive Airway Pressure (CPAP) device, noise generated from these devices is normally higher than that generated from the Non-positive type, and this limits their use in CPAP machines.

A.2 NON-POSITIVE TYPE AIR COMPRESSORS

Non-positive type air compressors are commonly called fans due to the relatively low air pressures achieved during operation. These compressors utilize the rotor to add kinetic energy to the air, resulting in an increase in pressure when the flow is partially decelerated at the exhaust port. Centrifugal one-stage fans do not require any form of liquid seal or lubrication, so they are well suited for supplying breathing quality air. However, they have relatively low output pressure due to internal air leakage and re-circulation within the rotor and shroud. With respect to the higher supply air pressure required for the CPAP system, the option of utilizing a multistage centrifugal fan as well as a regenerative blower is possible.

Due to the low airflow resistance encountered within the large diameter tube supplying the nasal mask, the low-pressure output is not a problem for the CPAP therapy devices. The model simulation presented in Chapter 3, however, predicts that a typical CPAP system will require a supply air pressure approximately 10 times greater than that generated by a commercial CPAP air delivery unit (ADU). Centrifugal fan performance predictions are necessary to ascertain if this method of air supply is capable of meeting the CPAP requirements.

Figure A-1 shows the performance characteristics of a typical commercially available centrifugal fan unit that meets the requirements of the CPAP system. This fan unit will supply an air volume flow rate that is well in excess of the 100 liters/min (3.5 SCFM) required by the CPAP system. However, it would additionally require some means by which the mass flow rate could be dynamically controlled. There is no data available on the control response of the fan unit, which could be used to regulate the pressure or mass flow.

A typical single stage CPAP fan consists of a centrifugal compressor that can generally be modeled as a rotodynamic device. The ADU

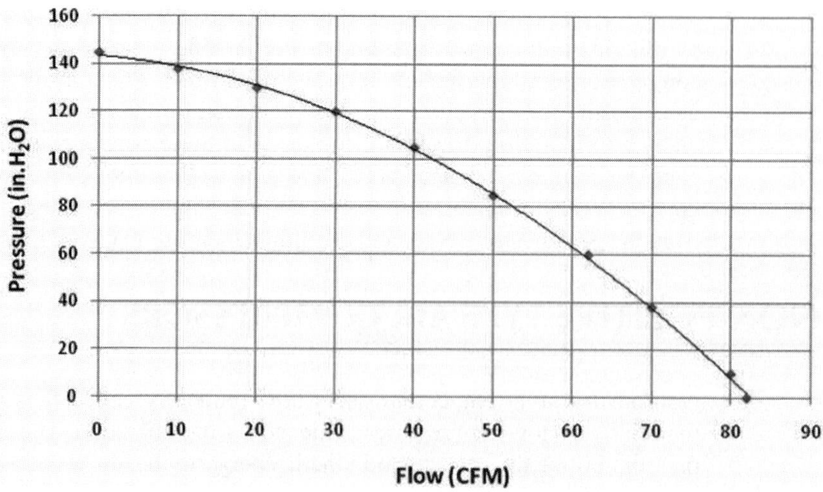

Figure A-1. Typical centrifugal compressor performance

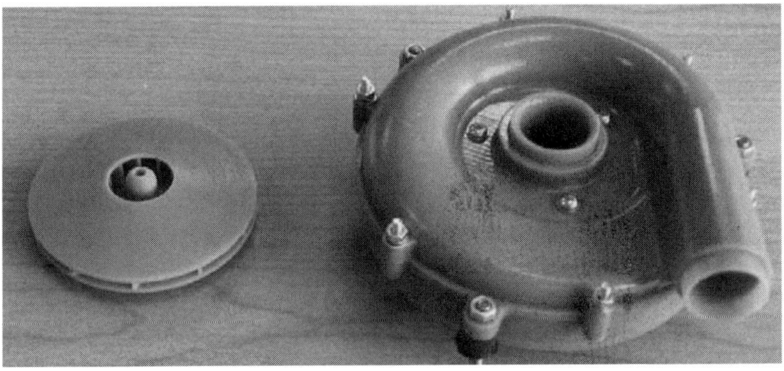

Figure A-2. ADU rotor and volute [Courtesy of Fisher & Paykel Healthcare Ltd]

device has to be able to produce high enough pressure to overcome the humidification reservoir, air delivery tube, and the mask in addition to the required pressure to treat the OSA, which is around 20 cm of water. If higher pressure is required at the ADU outlet, it can be achieved by either increasing the impeller diameter or the rotation speed. In either case, the rotational inertia would increase with the relationship:

$$I_{adu} = \omega_{adu}^2 \cdot r_{adu} \qquad (A-1)$$

where ω_{adu} and r_{adu} are the rotor speed and effective radius, respectively. CPAP manufacturers have developed various impellers, including blade angles and overall diameters depending on the specific applications of their devices. Figure A-2 shows typical rotor and volute designs for a CPAP device.

In addition to the rotor and volute, the type of brushless DC motor used for the ADU device differs between manufacturers. The impeller and volute designs differ significantly and would both result in different compressor efficiencies. Heat is added to the system as a result of compressor inefficiencies and in the form of heat produced from the driving DC motor. Figure A-3 shows a typical temperature rise-air volume flow rate for a CPAP compressor.

The inlet temperature is normally slightly higher as a result of localized heating of the air around the volute inside the ADU device. As the air gets heated by the ADU, its saturation vapor pressure increases but the absolute humidity of the air remains the same. As a result, the relative humidity (RH) of the air at the blower exit is lower than that at its inlet.

Higher air pressures from a centrifugal fan may still be attainable without the problem of utilizing a higher rotational speed or enlarged diameter through the use of multistage compression [2]. Based on the idealized assumption that each rotor stage will double the static air pressure, a five-stage compression will result in improving the commercial

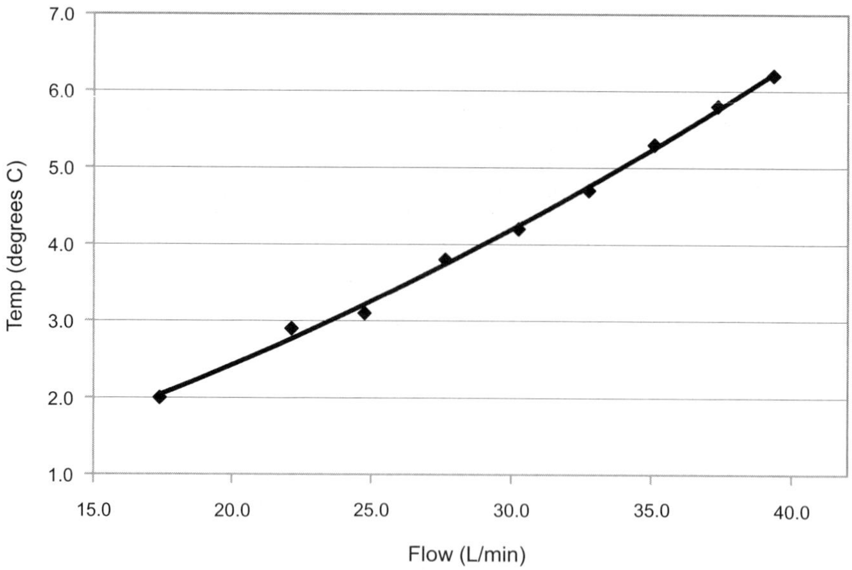

Figure A-3. Typical rise in air temperature between the inlet and outlet of the blower

fan unit to produce 185 cm H_2O of pressure. In practice, however, when the fan rotors are assembled in axial alignment on the same shaft, the airflow must turn 180° when passing between stages, resulting in lower efficiencies and hence lower air pressures. Furthermore, consideration must also be given to the air mass flow control, since the higher mass moment of inertia given by a multistage rotor would add to the delay in the ADU response to variation in mask pressure.

A possible alternative to a multistage centrifugal fan is the regenerative blower, also known as the vortex blower. This type of a single rotor fan unit produces a significantly higher static pressure when compared to the conventional centrifugal fan. However, it is characterized by a lower efficiency than that of a multistage centrifugal fan and produces higher noise levels due to increased turbulence.

REFERENCES

[1] Kishibuchi, A., Nosaka, M., and Fukanuma, T., Development of Continuous Running, Externally Controlled Variable Displacement Compressor. *SAE Transactions*, 1999. **108**(1): p. 1674–79.

[2] Bleier, F.P., *Fan Handbook: Selection, Application and Design*, 1998. McGraw-Hill, New York.

Appendix B

SENSORS USED IN CPAP

It is an advantage to operate the Continuous Positive Airway Pressure (CPAP) system at a lower pressure while monitoring the patient's airflow, and raise the pressure as the Obstructive Sleep Apnea (OSA) is detected, rather than maintain a fixed higher minimum pressure in order to reduce OSA symptoms. As explained in Chapter 5, controlling the mask pressure is an important feature that needs to be considered when a CPAP machine is developed. These features and other patient comfort conditions require the use of special types of air sensors. This appendix summarizes the basic concepts of airflow measurement methods that can be used to measure airflow rates within the air delivery tube or the mask. These methods and their operation mechanisms are discussed in the following sections and summarized in Table B-1.

B.1 DIGITAL PROPELLER ANEMOMETER

A propeller is normally located in the airflow stream, where the axial direction is coordinated (parallel) with the velocity direction of airflow. Assuming there is no friction and the rotational speed is linear relative to the velocity of airflow, the propeller rotation speed indicates the airflow velocity [1]. Each blade of a propeller rotates, passing a fixed point where electromagnetic induction or an optical couple enables the rate of the propeller rotation to be measured. Each running blade creates an electrical pulse when it passes the fixed point. The air velocity can be obtained indirectly by computing the amount of pulse in a set time period.

Commercially available fluid flow measurement range is from 0.01 to 5,000 m/min. The time constant is 2 to 10 ms. The higher the air velocity, the lower the time constant, and the device can be modeled as a first-order measuring system with a response time of 2 to 10 ms. The nonlinear error can be controlled between 0.05% of the design range (usually the rate of maximum and minimum value is 10:1). Usually, the output of

TABLE B-1. Several methods of airflow measurement

Principle	Operating Mechanism
Pressure	The pressure of flowing air varies with the velocity of air.
Pneumatics	Propeller can obtain power from flowing air to rotate; the rotational speed is proportional to the air velocity.
Lever	This air sensor has cantilevers and strain gauges fabricated at the bottom of sensory hairs. The output voltage was proportional to the velocity of air flow [8].
Heat lost	The rate of heat lost from probe corresponds to the air velocity.
Sound velocity	The difference between measured sound velocity and known sound velocity in steady air is proportional to the airflow velocity.
Corona ion deflection	Process of corona ion deflection in a gas flow together with proper electrode geometry.
Electromagnetic	The induced electromagnetic voltage of the coil varies with the speed of conductive fluid passing over the coil.

magnetic induction voltage is 10 mV to 100 mV. The output signal is of a square wave from digital pulses, which are displayed on a scope or interfaced to a microprocessor or computer. The accuracy of the propeller anemometer is lower than that found in a hot wire anemometer.

B.2 ELECTROMAGNETIC FLOW METER

This measurement device uses the principle of induction. When a conductor moves with a transverse velocity across a magnetic field, the positive charged particles of the conductor will be forced to move toward one end of the conductor and the negative charges to the other. Thus, a potential gradient is set up along the conductor, and there is a voltage difference between its two ends [2, 3]. A practical flow meter is contained within a stationary pipe, which must be nonmagnetic to allow the field to penetrate the fluid and is usually nonconductive, so that it does not provide a short-circuit path between the positive and negative induced potential at the fluid surface.

The main features of this device include: no flow obstruction in the tube, ability to measure reverse flows, insensitivity to fluid viscosity and density, and capability to measure rapid response to flow changes. However, these flow meters are appropriate only when using a conductive fluid or fluids containing conductive particles. Air is a non-conductive fluid and hence this device is not suitable for airflow measurement.

B.3 LASER DOPPLER ANEMOMETRY (LDA)

Using cylindrical lenses, a periodically pulsed laser beam is expanded into a two-dimensional "light sheet" defining a plane in the flow where velocity will be measured [4]. The light sheet is controlled by a spherical lens to about 1 mm thickness. Using a multiple-exposure method (like that utilized in a digital camera), the locations of the particles at two instants separated by a known time interval are used to compute the magnitude and direction of the particle's velocity, i.e., the air velocity.

LDA has a very high accuracy, but it is difficult to utilize for real-time applications and it is limited by needing near-neutrally-buoyant particles in the air. Complex instrument and high cost are other limitations.

B.4 HOT WIRE/FILM ANEMOMETER

Hot wire anemometers measure the air velocity by detecting the impact of velocity on heat transfer from a heated resistance wire located tangential to the airflow path [5]. Three types of electrical circuits are normally utilized with this device: constant voltage, constant current, and constant temperature circuits.

In a constant voltage or current hot wire/film sensor, a constant voltage or current is applied to the probe resistor. It is assumed that the value of the resistor does not vary with temperature and the generated heat is constant. The heat lost to the airflow is related to air velocity. Hence, it will cause a resistor temperature change that is proportional to the airflow velocity.

In a constant temperature hot wire/film sensor, where the probe resistor is kept at a constant temperature, the generated heat should be equal to the heat loss caused by the airflow. A driver circuit is used to control the power delivered to the heated resistor to keep the temperature at a constant value.

Constant voltage or current modes are rarely used due to the fact that if the fluid velocity drops rapidly, the heat loss will be much less than the generated heat, and it will cause the hot wire to quickly burn out. However, in the constant temperature mode, an anemometer uses the feedback circuit to self-balance the wire temperature.

Dependant on the different types of resistor material used, the thermal anemometers can be divided into hot wire and hot film. A hot film anemometer operates on the same principle as a hot wire anemometer; however, the metal wire resistor in a hot wire anemometer is replaced by a film resistor, which is supported on thin silicon beams [6]. The film resistor has higher and more reliable mechanical strength. This high mechanical strength prevents distortion of the film, thus preventing a drop in the accuracy of measurement.

One main limitation of the thermal anemometer is that it cannot identify reversed airflow because of its working principle, hence it is not suitable for turbulent air measurments. Thermal anemometers have a limited lower range of measurement due to the convective heat loss from the wire [7]. Heat generation and heat loss will cause time delay in real-time meaurement. This effect is significant in high frequency dynamic measurement, such as the type encounted in the automotive industry. In this application the airflow sensor itself has a response delay, resulting in the measured amount of air becoming inconsistent with the amount of air flowing into the cylinders due to the time delay [8].

Because of the variation of ambient and air temperatures, the temperature compensation of a thermal anemometer will directly affect the accuracy of measurement. This problem can be solved by fabricating two symmetical probe resistors in the circuit. One of the probes is heated via its resistor by means of a control circuit, while the other probe is unheated and serves as an ambient temperature reference for temperature compensation. The average temperature of each probe is reflected in the temperature-dependent resistance of its nickel film [8].

The thermal anemometer circuit obtains an output by detecting the relative temperature difference between the heated probe and a reference probe. When the ambient air temperature rises, not only does the temperature of the heated probe elevate, but also that of the reference probe. This leads to no net difference in probe temperature, and the measurement of air velocity is not affected by the fluctuation of ambient temperature. A temperature compensation circuit is normally designed to maintain a constant ratio between the resistance of the heated probe and the sum of the temperature reference and temperature compensation resistances. This ratio is typically selected to maintain the heated element at about 180°C above ambient, in order to burn off any oil and water deposits that might otherwise condense on the hot film and affect its heat transfer characteristics.

In order to get the temperature value of probes, the instantaneous temperature of each probe is determined by the temperature-dependent resistance of its nickel film [8]. The most suitable planar Negative Temperature Coefficient (NTC) thermistor geometry for an air sensor is a segmented type with an optimized surface value of 75 × 12 × 0.5 mm. It is used to cover part of an open air gauge and conduct heat from flowing air. The resistivity difference obtained on the thermistors is compared with the volume velocity of air laminar flow at room ambient temperature and humidity [7].

Accuracy and Measurement Range

Previous experiments have proven that airflow can be measured within 0.5% deviation [8]. A micromachined, monolithic silicon mass-airflow sensor has been developed for measuring engine intake airflow in the range of 1 to 60 m/s. It has a response time of under 1 ms (600 μs) and can be temperature compensated to a deviation of ±3.5% error or less in indicated flow over a temperature range of –30°C to +40°C. The device can withstand bombardment by particles up to 50 μm in size in the airstream, or larger ones if elements with reduced accuracy are used [6].

B.5 ULTRASONIC ANEMOMETER

The ultrasonic anemometer measures the average velocity of flow over the path that the sound wave propagates [9]. The measurement principle is based on the linear relationship between the inverse Transit Time Difference (TTD, which is the time difference between the sound wave traveling along one direction in a constant distance and that along the inverse direction) and the air velocity [5].

Another type of a sensor based on the TTD uses one transmitter and one receiver, both placed along the airflow path. An alternative is to have another sensor based on utilizing an inverse TTD, by using a pair of transmitters and an opposing a pair of receivers, placed along the airflow path. The sound wave from the transmitter delivered to the flow stream is sent to the receiver downstream and vice versa. The time difference of sound wave propagation is proportional to the average air velocity over the path between the transmitter and the receiver [9]. There are two types of ultrasonic waves generated from the transmitter: the first is called a pulsed type ultrasonic anemometer, which determines the velocity by measuring the inverse TTD of two pulses along a known path; the second is called a continuous wave ultrasonic anemometer, which is based on the same principle as the pulsed type, but instead it utilizes a continuous wave [5].

Ultrasonic anemometers avoid the need of temperature compensation over a wide temperature range. The TTD ultrasonic anemometer has a high dynamic range, good linearity, and very low dead band [10]. Ultrasonic anemometers have faster response speed than other anemometers, such as the propeller type, and lack any moving parts [5]; however, they need a microprocessor to generate ultrasonic waves and also to compute propagated time.

Accuracy and Measurement Range

The ultrasonic anemometer is able to measure wind velocity in the horizontal plane in a range from 0 to about 100 km/h, with a dead band of 2 cm/s and an accuracy better than 3% in a temperature range from –25 to +75 °C [10]. Previous experimentation has shown that when an air velocity of 0.4 m/s is measured by the ultrasonic anemometer, a simulation gives a theoretical value of 0.3951 m/s with an error of 0.0049 m/s (1.2%). Engineers have simulated velocities from 0 to 2.0 m/s, which have produced a linear relationship between air velocity and ultrasonic path time [5].

B.6 SUMMARY

A summary analysis of the several methods of airflow measurement techniques required, along with their advantages and limitations for the

CPAP system, are listed in Table B-2. Several aspects are considered to determine the suitability of the airflow sensor to the CPAP system with respect to measurable range, sensitivity, response time, suitable dimension to locate the probe with the CPAP machine, and reasonable cost. Recent technological developments of have enabled the ultrasonic transceiver to become much smaller and cheaper than before, and this makes it possible for application in the CPAP system. However, there are some limitations to the ultrasonic airflow measuring method in the CPAP system, including the fact that these sensors can only be located in the inlet channel of the CPAP machine and are very difficult to locate in other positions, such as the outlet of a blower, humidifier, tube, and mask, as they need the transducers to be positioned a specific distance apart along the airflow path. Within the air inlet channel, the two transceivers are not suitable to be fixed at corners as the air turbulence at these locations is very complex. If the transceivers are located near the middle of the airflow track, it will increase the airflow resistance slightly, but will lead to better accuracy of results.

TABLE B-2. Summary comparison of airflow sensors

Methods	Advantages	Limitations for CPAP
Propeller	Large range (0.01 to 15,000 ft3/min) High accuracy Fast response: 2 to 10 ms	Large dimensions Low sensitivity Mechanical corruption
Electromagnetic	No flow obstruction Wide linear range Acceptable accuracy Rapid response time Insensitivity to viscosity and density	Require conductive fluid or including conductive particles in the fluid High cost
Laser doppler anemometry	Very large range Very high accuracy Suitable for record flow traces	Not good for real-time applications Need near-neutrally-buoyant particles Complex instruments Very high cost
Pitot-static tube	Small error: 0.46% Large range: 0 to 4.33 m/s Low cost	Limited response speed Large dimensions Accuracy is affected by many factors
Thermal hot wire/film	Proper range: 1 to 60 m/s Low deviation Small dimension probe Low cost	Response time depends on probe size Accuracy is affected by ambient temperature
Ultrasonic	Large range High accuracy (<3% error) Adapt in extremes of temperature and humidity Fast response (<3 ms)	Complicated setup High cost

REFERENCES

[1] Saad, N.H., Janin, Z., and Sahab, A.R.M. Instrumentation of Digital-Propeller-Anemometer, 2003. AsiaSense 2003 Asian Conference on Sensors. p. 341–5.

[2] Bennion, D., Electromagnetic Flowmeters for Difficult Media, 1992. "Chem Engr. Issue (516): p. 33.

[3] Zbinden, M., Electromagnetic Flowmeters, 1987. Electricite de France, Bulletin de la Direction des Etudes et Recherches, Serie A: Nucleaire, Hydr. Issue (4): p. 51.

[4] Doebelin, E.O., Measurement Systems: Application and Design, 5th Ed., 2004, McGraw Hill. p. 103–214, 578–672.

[5] Tang, S., Federspiel, C.C., and Auslander, D.M., Pulsed Type Ultrasonic Anemometer Based on a Double FFT Procedure, 2003. Proceedings of IEEE Sensors, Institute of Electrical and Electronics Engineers Inc., Toronto, Ont., Canada. Vol. 2: p. 326–31.

[6] Stephan, C.H., and Zanini, M., A Micromachined, Silicon Mass-air-flow Sensor for Automotive Applications, 1991. International Conference on Solid-State Sensors and Actuators, Digest of Technical Papers, TRANSDUCERS '91. p. 30–3.

[7] Aleksic, O.S., Nikolic, P.M., Lukovic, D., Savic, S., Pejovic, V.Z., and Radojcic, B.M., A Thick Film NTC Thermistor Air Flow Sensor, 2004. 24th International Conference on Microelectronics. Vol. 1: p. 185–8.

[8] Takahashi, S., and Sekozawa, T., Air-fuel Ratio Control in Gasoline Engines Based on State Estimation and Prediction Using Dynamic Models, 1995. Proceedings of the 1995 IEEE IECON 21st International Conference on Industrial Electronics, Control, and Instrumentation. Vol. 1: p. 217–27.

[9] Teerawatanachai, S., Komiya, K., and Sasamoto, H., Estimating the Velocity Profile of Air Flow by Means of the Ultrasonic Translation Time Computed Tomography Method, 1991. Vol. 3: p. 2379–84.

[10] Aprilesi, G.C., De Cicco, G., and Taroni, A., A Microprocessor-Based, Three Axes, Ultrasonic Anemometer, 1983. Ultrasonics Symposium, p. 295–8.

INDEX

Page numbers followed by *f* and *t* indicate figures and tables, respectively.